THE SYMPTOM ICEBERG

THE SYMPTOM ICEBERG

A study of community health

DAVID RAINSFORD HANNAY

ROUTLEDGE & KEGAN PAUL
London, Boston and Henley

First published in 1979
by Routledge & Kegan Paul Ltd
39 Store Street,
London WC1E 7DD,
Broadway House,
Newtown Road,
Henley-on-Thames,
Oxon RG9 1EN and
9 Park Street,
Boston, Mass. 02108, USA
Printed in Great Britain by
Redwood Burn Ltd
Trowbridge and Esher

British Library Cataloguing in Publication Data

Hannay, David Rainsford
  The symptom iceberg.
  1. Woodside Health Centre 2. Semiology
  3. Diseases - Reporting - Scotland -
  Glasgow 4. Social medicine - Scotland -
  Glasgow
  1. Title
  362.1'2   RC69   78-41166

ISBN 0 7100 8982 1

For Janet,
Mark, Neil, and Stephen

CONTENTS

ILLUSTRATIONS

(All figures have been corrected to the nearest whole number, except for Table 8.1, Figure 9.3 and Appendix II which were corrected to one decimal place, and the tables in Appendix V which were corrected to three places of decimals.)

ACKNOWLEDGMENTS

This study was made possible by a research grant from the Social Science Research Council, and by the help of E. J. Maddox as research assistant, and Mrs Elizabeth McLaren, Mrs Helen Scobbie, and Mrs Margaret Wyllie as interviewers. My debt to them is considerable.

The research was carried out while I held a joint appointment in the Departments of Social and Economic Research, and Community Medicine at the University of Glasgow; and this book was written from the Department of General Practice in Glasgow. I am grateful to Professor T. Anderson and the late Professor Donald Robertson for allowing the project to start, to Professor L. C. Hunter and Professor G. T. Stewart for enabling it to continue, and to Professor J. H. Barber for encouraging its completion. Inevitably, many people have made helpful suggestions, especially members of the above departments; in particular the assistance of E. J. Maddox and encouragement of Dr V. M. Hawthorne are gratefully acknowledged, as well as the constructive comments of Professor L. C. Hunter.

My thanks are also due to Dr Fiona Williams, Mrs Sue Farbman, and Andrew Sweeney for assistance with computing, to David McLaren and Keith Wilson-Davis for advice on statistics, to Mrs Julie Handle and Andrew Wyllie for help with post-coding, and to the following for their patience with the typing involved: Mrs Moira Dougan, Miss Isobel McKnight, Mrs Winifred Marshall, Miss Morley Burns, Mrs Margaret Steele, and Mrs Marian Robertson.

This study would not have been possible without the cooperation and understanding of the General Practitioners at the Woodside Health Centre, who kindly gave permission for their patients to be interviewed. I would also like to thank the many people in Glasgow who allowed us into their homes, and answered our questions. It is hoped that the results may in some way repay the privilege of their confidence and courtesy.

In addition, grateful acknowledgments are due to Dr Hope for permission to adapt material from his 'Symptom Sign Inventory' published by Hodder & Stoughton; and to Professor H. J. Eysenck for permission to include questions from the shorter Maudsley Personality Inventory.

Chapter 1

INTRODUCTION

'Statistical connotes an inquiry into the state of the country for
the purpose of ascertaining the quantum of happiness enjoyed by its
inhabitants and the means of its future improvement.'

Sir John Sinclair (1754 - 1835)

BACKGROUND

This study is based on 1,344 home interviews of patients registered
with doctors practising from a new health centre in Glasgow. The
main objectives were to assess the prevalence of symptoms and
patterns of referral in the community, and to explore factors which
might be associated with these, such as personal characteristics,
the environment, and people's perception of their symptoms and the
services available.

The aims of the study were primarily descriptive, rather than
being concerned with proving or disproving particular theories.
Indeed one of the problems of our present knowledge in this area is
that research often tends to prejudge the issues involved. This
may be because questions are asked from a particular point of view,
which may be subjective. Another reason is the tendency for social
science to start from 'a priori' hypotheses which may restrict and
limit enquiry, when so often we do not even know the relevant
questions to ask. The basis of all scientific endeavour must be a
clear description of what is happening, and this may be hampered by
forcing the data into preconceived theories. Unlike the natural
sciences, it is not usually possible to experiment in social science.
It is therefore often appropriate to allow the accurate description
of situations with associated factors to point the way towards
causal explanations, without necessarily first postulating discrete
hypotheses. Such an approach will inevitably cut across the boundaries of academic disciplines, which themselves tend to impose the
constraints of particular perspectives.

For a study which is primarily descriptive it is important to
present the facts and findings as clearly and concisely as possible,
and hence the extensive use of figures in this book as well as
tables. It is also important to state clearly how the results were

achieved, and therefore the methods used have been included as an integral part of the text. Because the approach is broad and impinges on many different areas of interest, the findings have been placed in the context of current concepts and related studies, although there is not the space to discuss all of these in detail. The need for a descriptive study of this sort is emphasized by the conflicting findings of current research, the apparent inadequacy of social theory, and the practical changes taking place in the provision of services. These are discussed below, and a more ecological approach is indicated which will be returned to at the end of the book when considering the theoretical implications of the results.

Current research indicates a considerable lack of fit between the recipients and providers of services. For instance, morbidity studies suggest that there is a large amount of ill health in the community which does not reach medical attention.(1) The size of this illness 'iceberg' depends on whether presymptomatic conditions are included, but symptom surveys carried out recently in countries with very different primary care systems,(2) or in the United Kingdom both before (3) and after the introduction of the National Health Service,(4) all indicate that about three-quarters of the population have symptoms at any one time, but only one-quarter will be attending doctors.

These findings do not fit in with studies of British general practice,(5) which show that many doctors complain about being bothered with 'trivia' which do not require their medical skills. There appears to be a conflict of expectations between family doctors and patients, with many people going to doctors when perhaps they need not do so, whereas others do not go when they probably should.

From a theoretical point of view sociology has not provided a perspective which accounts for these conflicting findings. A functional approach in terms of the 'sick role' with rights and obligations, as put forward by Talcott Parsons,(6) does not explain what appears to be happening. Nor do concepts based on doctor-patient interaction (7) provide an adequate basis for the observed variations in the ways in which people do or do not refer themselves.

At the time this research was being carried out considerable changes were taking place in the organization of services in Scotland. First, surgeries belonging to individual partnerships were being replaced in Glasgow by purpose-built health centres. The survey was based on one of the first of these health centres to open in Glasgow, containing eight practices with twenty doctors, covering over 40,000 patients. The second change to take place was the advent of social work departments.(8) As a major part of the so-called 'trivia' about which doctors complain appears to involve social problems,(9) it seemed necessary to extend the definition of symptoms beyond the physical to those which were mental and social. It also seemed appropriate to include social workers as possible sources of professional referral.

The project was not, however, an attempt to evaluate any particular form of service such as health centres or social work departments, since such an attempt would require before-and-after studies, or the use of control groups. Inevitably the results throw some light on people's perceptions and use of these new facilities, but

only as part of a total picture of the extent to which services fit
community needs as defined by symptoms. Because everyone in the
United Kingdom should officially be registered with a General
Practitioner, the health centre records were used primarily as a
convenient sampling frame, as well as a means of introduction via
the General Practitioner. The majority of those interviewed were
not under any treatment at the time and some had never been to the
health centre. The accuracy of these records was therefore of some
importance for the provision of community services as well as for
the research sample.

The extent to which services fit the needs of communities in a
essence involves two levels of adaptation. First, the referral
behaviour of individuals in response to perceived symptoms, and
second, the response of society in terms of the provision of
services. Information about the former is essential as a continuing feedback if there is to be effective adaptation by the latter.
In broader terms such research is concerned with the coping
behaviour of individuals who are self-aware and continually adapting
to their environment. Nowhere are environmental factors more
sharply defined than in Glasgow, which has the highest indices of
urban deprivation in the British Isles,(10) and possibly in
Europe. In addition, the Clydeside conurbation has high mortality
rates for the common afflictions of the Western world, such as
ischaemic heart disease and lung cancer.(11) And yet the medical
profession in Scotland has an international reputation, and it was
the first part of the United Kingdom to set up social work departments. The evidence suggests a failure of that adaptation which is
a prerequisite of health,(12) and often of survival. This maladaptation is not just of individuals but also of society, which itself
has a coping behaviour, for it is a premise of sociology that
society can also be studied in a sense as a behaving organism.
Sociology itself is evidence of that organism's self-awareness, and
the provision of medical care and social services are examples of
its coping behaviour.

The threshold of awareness at which an individual or society
starts to adapt is balanced in the scales of acceptance on the one
hand and anxiety on the other. The factors which tip the scales
are complex and may be very different for an individual and for the
society in which he lives. But for the adaptations of both individual and society to be effective, they should at least correspond.
The evidence suggests that they do not do so closely, and an
analysis of the factors involved might lead to clearer concepts
about what is happening, and have implications for the provision of
services such as primary medical care and social work.

The aims of the study were therefore primarily concerned with
describing what was going on in the community in terms of symptoms
and what people did about them. Measures of symptom prevalence and
referral behaviour were defined, such as the extent of the symptom
'iceberg' and 'trivia'. Relationships were then explored between
these measures and factors such as personal characteristics, the
environment, and the subjects' perceptions of their symptoms and
the services available. Such an approach is inductive in that it
starts from the basis of recorded facts about symptoms and referral
behaviour, rather than deductively trying to prove or disprove

particular theories.   No assumptions were made about the definition
of sickness, because symptoms are subjective without necessarily
implying ill health, and referral is the action taken about a symptom
which may include doing nothing at all.

DATA COLLECTION

The data for the study were collected by home interviews using a
coded questionnaire which is shown in Appendix I.   Emphasis was
placed on confidentiality and no name or address appeared on the
folders.   Each subject was given a four-figure number, the first
digit of which indicated the interviewer.   Most questions were coded
directly by the interviewer in coding boxes down the right-hand
margin of the questionnaire, except those questions marked with an
asterisk which were open-ended and coded afterwards (post-coded).
   The questions on symptoms were in four main groups and referred
to the previous two weeks only.(13)   The first group was for
physical symptoms and consisted of forty-four questions most of
which included three or four related symptoms.   These questions were
intended to be mutually exclusive and exhaustive, and were asked of
all subjects except for a few which were only relevant to a particular sex or age-group (e.g. post-menopausal bleeding).   Where
medical conditions were wholly or partly defined in terms of
symptoms, the appropriate methodology was used, for instance for
chronic bronchitis,(14) and heart disease.(15)   All the questions
were phrased in simple non-technical language and referred to things
people might have noticed about themselves, rather than to diseases.
   Symptoms are by definition subjective, and no attempt was made
at objective evaluation or diagnosis.   Nor was there any feedback to
a medical source because of confidentiality.   In view of this,
symptoms which might be dangerous, such as painless bleeding, were
marked (D) in the questionnaire so that the interviewer could advise
the person to see a doctor.   Any positive physical symptom was
graded by the respondent for pain, disability, perceived seriousness,
duration, and referral, according to the grading scale codes on the
left-hand cover of the questionnaire.   The appropriate two-figure
code was then entered directly into the coding boxes provided in
the margin for each symptom, as indicated at the top of the grading-
scale sheets.   The same scales were used for adult mental symptoms
and children's behavioural symptoms as were used for physical
symptoms, but a simpler scale for worry or inconvenience was used
for social symptoms in adults, for which the referral was post-coded.
All these grading scales for symptoms recorded the subjective
replies of the respondents themselves, and no objective assessments
about symptoms or referral were made by the interviewers.
   The second group of questions was for mental symptoms.   These
were asked of adults only and were adapted from the Foulds Symptom
Sign Inventory.(16)   This was designed as a psychiatric screening
questionnaire and each question had been validated against subsequent diagnoses.   The most predictive symptoms for each diagnosis
were chosen and grouped into eight main questions.   No single symptom
by itself was highly diagnostic, but taken as a whole, a number of
positive responses was likely to indicate psychiatric disturbance.

The third group of questions related to behavioural symptoms for children of 15 years or under. These included the main developmental milestones, and covered those kinds of behaviour which the Department of Child Psychiatry in Glasgow had found to be the commonest presenting symptoms at their clinic.(17)   For children all the questions, including physical symptoms, were asked of a parent or other adult present about the child. The questionnaire branched so that the behavioural symptoms for children were asked instead of questions about mental or social symptoms.

The fourth group of questions was for social symptoms, which were asked of adults only. There were four main questions concerning difficulties with children or teenagers, difficulties with other relations, financial difficulties, and other problems with day-to-day life. These broad categories were formulated from the commonest reasons for clients presenting for social case work at a family centre in Glasgow.(18)   The questions were open-ended and graded more simply than the physical, mental and behavioural symptoms, all of which were considered together as medical symptoms for analysis, as opposed to social symptoms which were graded separately for worry or inconvenience.

The interview commenced with sociographic information about age, sex, marital status, occupation, education, religion, housing, and mobility. Occupation was post-coded into social class,(19) and the length of formal schooling rather than qualification was used for education.(20)   A distinction was made between purely nominal religious allegiance, and active participation, which was defined as attending a religious function at least once a month.   The questions on housing were partly based on methodology developed by the Scottish Development Department,(21) and mobility was assessed in terms of length of residence, number of moves, as well as place of birth and upbringing.

The questions on symptoms were preceded by information about past medical history, together with a short self-assessment of present health, which acted as a check on the symptoms elicited by subsequent questioning. The list of symptoms was followed by questions on the use and perception of medical services and social work, together with information about medicine taking, family planning, and smoking habits. The questionnaire ended with respondents' comments about the interview, and final assessments by the interviewer.

For those of 15 years or under, the sociographic and symptom data referred to the child, but questions on the use and perception of services were asked of all respondents whether answering for themselves or a child. This also applied to the personality and intelligence tests which were the only parts of the questionnaire to be self-completed. The personality test was adapted from the shorter Maudsley Personality Inventory (22) using phrasing which had been found to be more applicable to Glasgow.(23)   The intelligence questions were taken from one of the shorter 16 PF personality tests.(24)   These methodologies were used because the tests were short, easy to administer, and had been widely used for comparability and standardization.

The questionnaire was tested in a pilot study for feasibility, acceptability, and length of time taken for an interview, which in

the main survey was an average of 36 minutes. In general the
interviewers were well received and it was often more difficult to
stop the respondents talking, than to encourage them to start. In
this respect some interviews fulfilled a therapeutic function, quite
apart from the collection of data.

Random monthly samples, without replacement, were drawn from the
health centre's computer file during the course of a calendar year.
This allowed for a steady rate of interviewing and took account of
the continual population changes due to births, deaths, and mobility.
The total sample size was estimated from the assumed accuracy of the
practice lists,(25,26) and the expected proportion of the main
dependent variables.(27) In the event the addresses on the computer
file were less accurate than expected,(28) so that surplus names had
to be drawn each month.

Five interviewers took part in the survey, and each address was
visited with a letter of introduction which was handed personally
to the subject, so that contact was established and any queries
could be answered. The introduction was via the family doctor and
the reasons for, and the nature of, the survey were explained.
Confidentiality was stressed, with the fact that no information
could be passed on, and therefore no return visit was possible after
the interview.

Subjects were either interviewed at the first contact or an
appointment arranged. If necessary up to two return calls were
made in the evenings or at weekends, when the person was thought to
be at the address but out at the time. If the subject was not at
the address given then the reasons were noted. All the interviewers
had previous experience of such work and were carefully briefed,
both before and during the survey.

RESPONSE

The response to the survey was determined by the accuracy of the
sampling frame and the reactions of individual respondents. This
first factor is considered in some detail, not only because of the
implications for research bias, but because the quality of address
registration is of fundamental importance for the provision of
community services, especially in a reorganized and supposedly
integrated health service. The response of individual subjects
indicates the acceptability of the survey, which is relevant in
view of the subjective nature of the data.

The overall response is shown in Figure 1.1. Out of 3,414
addresses visited during the year, 54 per cent of subjects were at
the address given, and a total of 1,344 (40 per cent) interviews
were carried out, representing 3.1 per cent of the mean list size
during the year. For those not at the address given, an attempt
was made to find out what had happened to the person concerned.
Many had moved or never been heard of, reflecting the high rate of
mobility in central Glasgow, much of it due to rehousing and slum
clearance. This last factor is shown by the number of addresses
where the house was found to be demolished or derelict.

The redevelopment of older property in city centres typically
results in a high rate of mobility, and one study using health

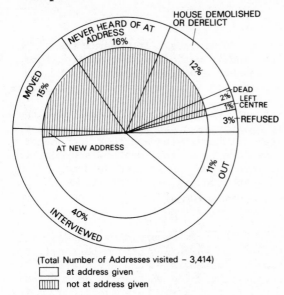

(Total Number of Addresses visited – 3,414)

☐ at address given

▥ not at address given

FIGURE 1.1   Overall response

service records estimated that internal migration in Scotland approaches 25 per cent of the population per year.(29) The situation is exacerbated in Glasgow by the high proportion of public housing, much of it being renewed, and by the tendency of corporation tenants to move because of rent arrears, which had more than doubled in the two years preceding the survey.(30)

The destination of those who had moved was recorded for the first six months of interviewing,(28) and it was found that over one-third had moved elsewhere in the Glasgow area, and were therefore still likely to be registered with their doctor at the health centre. No information was available for most of the remainder, but about a quarter of those who had moved were known to be living away from Glasgow, and therefore could not effectively be registered at the health centre.

During the course of the year about three-quarters of the computer file was updated, but this made little difference to the accuracy of the monthly samples as shown in Figure 1.2. It seemed that these changes were merely keeping the accurate part of the file up to date, but were making little impression on the inaccurate part. In fact the size of the official executive council lists for the health centre was about 38,000, compared to approximately 44,000 on the computer file. The difference just about accounts for those who were no longer in the Glasgow area as estimated from the information about those who had moved.

Although births, deaths, and changes of doctor should officially be registered with the executive council, there is no way of routinely recording changes of address within an executive council area. This could only be recorded when someone attended the health centre, where the checking of addresses became increasingly routine. As there is no policy of statutory address registration in Britain, it was not possible to trace the non-responders, and some of those drawn in the sample were found to have moved or been

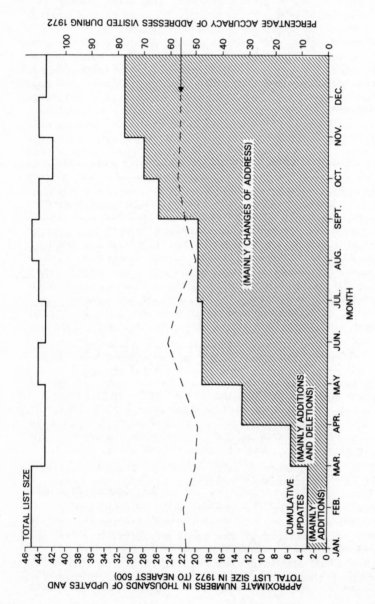

FIGURE 1.2   Computer file

dead for several years. Other studies have shown considerable
inaccuracies in executive council lists in Scotland,(25,26) but it
is likely that those who should not have been registered were
balanced by those who should have been, so that there was no overall
inflation of the doctors' lists as far as the official executive
council lists were concerned.

Those who were not at the address given would tend to be frequent
movers, who were under-utilizers of medical care. Attempts were
therefore made to compare the available data on those not at the
addresses given with those who were. It was found that both males
and females between 16 and 44 years old were the least likely to be
at the addresses given for them, presumably because of the greater
mobility and comparative health of these age-groups.

There were considerable differences in the accuracy of the eight
practice lists at the health centre. Those practices which had a
high proportion of patients in areas of redevelopment were the most
inaccurate, with more non-responders for whom the address was found
to be demolished or derelict. By assigning a six-figure 100-metre-
square grid reference to each address it was possible to produce
computer maps showing the distribution of accurate and inaccurate
addresses. As can be seen from Figures 1.3 a and b almost all the
health centre patients lived north of the river Clyde, with a tendency to cluster along the line of the main Maryhill Road, where many
of the practices had lock-up surgeries before moving to the health
centre. The maps show the extent to which this concentration had
been dispersed by slum clearance in the centre, and rehousing in
large peripheral estates.

Non-responders at the address given tended either to be adults
of working age who were the most likely to be out, or the elderly
who were the most likely to refuse. The biggest single factor in
refusal appeared to be ill health, which implies that the amount of
acute or serious illness found during the survey was an underest-
imate, especially as some of those who were out were in hospital.

Although the proportion of patients drawn from each practice
corresponded closely to the total proportion on the computer file,
the numbers actually interviewed depended on the accuracy of the
practice lists. Exactly the same number of interviews were done
each month - namely 122 - during 1972, partly to maintain a steady
rate of data collection and partly to look at any seasonal variations in symptoms and referral patterns. In fact, the dependent
variables for symptom frequency and referral behaviour did not show
a significant correlation with either practice or month, although
individual symptoms, such as those of respiratory illness, might
well have done so.

Most people had no comments to make about the interview after it
was over. Of those who expressed a definite opinion the great
majority were favourable, and only 2.5 per cent were critical in
some way. A few did not like the intelligence test and others
thought the interview too long, or objected to questions on religion,
family planning, or personality. The great majority, however, were
not only pleased to help, but were interested in the results.
Several said they found the interview helpful in giving them a
chance to talk about their problems to someone who was prepared to
listen.

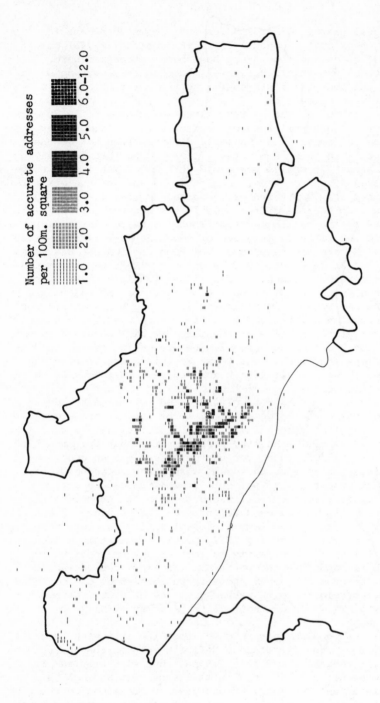

FIGURE 1.3a Map of accurate addresses

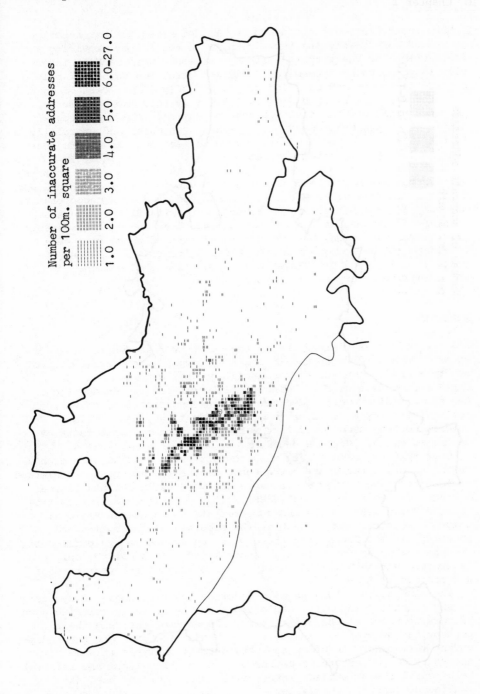

FIGURE 1.3b Map of inaccurate addresses

Many interviews were conducted in crowded homes against a background of both family and television, with the latter providing a distraction for the former. Although attempts were made to interview respondents by themselves, this was often impossible if only because there was nowhere else to go, and only 41 per cent of subjects were interviewed alone. Inevitably this made the more personal questions difficult to ask and answer. The most frequent single other person present was a parent or spouse, and especially in the latter case there was likely to be reticence about subjects such as family or marital problems.

Most respondents were very helpful, and only a few were uncooperative once they had agreed to being interviewed. In less than 2 per cent did the interviewers think that subjects had been uncooperative and only 4 per cent were rated as poor for reliability. These subjective assessments at the end of the interview showed considerable interviewer variation, but the great majority of those seen were considered to be cooperative and reliable informants. As one 35-year-old unemployed bricklayer commented, 'I'm glad someone is bothering; it's very interesting.'

ANALYSIS

All the addresses visited during the survey were coded to 100-metre-squares on a grid reference in order to compare the distribution of accurate and inaccurate addresses by computer mapping using the CAMAP system developed at Edinburgh University.(31) In addition the names visited were coded for age, sex and practice, as well as for whether they were interviewed and if not, why not. This information was used to compare responders with non-responders as described in the previous section.

Data from the main survey questionnaire were punched onto eighty column cards, after post-coding where necessary, and then transferred to computer tape. The results were analysed using the Statistical Package for Social Sciences (SPSS) (32) via on-line facilities from Glasgow University to the IBM computer at the Edinburgh Regional Computing Centre. As a check on the accuracy of the coding and punching, it was found that there were ten errors in the print-out for the number of interviews done per month. This was the only pre-determined variable in the survey and represented an error rate of 0.7 per cent.

The aims of the study were to describe the prevalence of symptoms in the community and what people did about them, in relation to such factors as personal characteristics, the environment, and their perceptions of symptoms and services. These factors were the independent variables. In order to carry out the analysis it was necessary to convert the measures of symptom prevalence and referral behaviour for each subject into scores which could be used as continuous dependent variables.

Frequency distributions of all the variables were first obtained, before the dependent variables for symptom prevalence and referral behaviour were computed as described below. The independent sociographic variables were recoded where necessary, to give categories of reasonable size and to assign missing values. The measures of

symptom prevalence and referral behaviour were then broken down as
continuous variables to give their mean values for each category of
the independent variables, and also cross-tabulated in a grouped
form with the independent variables. The significance of the breakdown results were tested by an analysis of variance,(33,34) and the
chi-squared test was used to test the significance of the cross-
tabulations.(32,35)

In order to compute the referral scores the types of referral
were first graded into a ranking scale of 1 for no referral, 2 for
an informal or lay referral, and 3 for a formal or professional
referral. A lay referral was an informal referral to a relative,
friend or acquaintance which did not primarily involve a professional
role, as opposed to a formal professional referral. For the purposes of computing referral scores, physical, mental and behavioural
symptoms were considered together as medical symptoms, in contrast
to social symptoms for which different grading scales were used.
Social symptoms that were said to cause no worry or inconvenience
were excluded from the referral scores.

Of the large number of possible correlations between the 10 computed dependent variables and 87 independent variables, just over
one-quarter were significant at the 0.05 level. Multivariate
analysis was therefore carried out for each dependent variable with
the object of gaining some perspective on the relative importance
of the independent variables, rather than testing specific hypotheses.
Only those independent variables that might be causal and that were
at least ranking scales or could be transformed into dummy variables
(27) were employed in SPSS programmes for multiple regression.

In fact only a small proportion of the variation of any of the
dependent variables was accounted for by the independent variables
in regression analysis. This was perhaps not surprising in view of
the complex nature of the dependent variables which were synthesizing computations from the initial data. In addition, multivariate analysis of this kind stretches the quality of the information by assuming interval scales and linear relationships, unless
special adjustments are made.

The analysis could be likened to a stepwise pyramid based on
data about the prevalence of symptoms and referral together with
sociographic information concerning the subjects involved. From
this descriptive base ten dependent variables were calculated, as
shown in Figure 1.4. These dependent variables converted the
detailed data on symptoms, including grading scales and referrals
for each symptom, into single scores for each person. As the
average number of symptoms per subject was about 5, with a maximum
of 25, the dependent variables represented a considerable simplification. Inevitably, much specific information about individual
symptoms was left behind in the process, although there were four
separate scores for the number of symptoms per person, representing
the broad categories of physical, mental, behavioural and social
symptoms.

The other six dependent variables related to referral behaviour.
They defined numerical scores for patterns of referral using the
grading scales for individual symptoms. As the grading scales for
social symptoms were different from those used for physical, mental
or behavioural symptoms, those latter were combined as medical

---

SYMPTOM PREVALENCE

1   Number of physical symptoms per person

2   Number of mental symptoms per adult

3   Number of behavioural symptoms per child

4   Number of social symptoms per adult

TENDENCY TO REFER FORMALLY

5   Mean medical referral score $= \dfrac{\text{sum of medical referral gradings}}{\text{number of medical symptoms}}$

6   Mean social referral score $= \dfrac{\text{sum of social referral gradings}}{\text{number of social symptoms}}$

SYMPTOM 'ICEBERG'

7   Incongruous medical lay referral score = Number of medical symptoms per person for which the referral was none or lay, when either the pain or disability was severe or the symptom was considered to be serious.

8   Incongruous social lay referral score = Number of social symptoms per adult for which the referral was none or lay, when the worry or inconvenience was severe.

SYMPTOM 'TRIVIA'

9   Incongruous medical professional referral score = Number of medical symptoms per person for which the referral was professional, when both pain and disability were none and the symptom was not thought to be serious.

10 Incongruous social professional referral score = Number of social symptoms per adult for which the referral was professional when the worry or inconvenience was slight.

THESE 10 DEPENDENT VARIABLES WERE DERIVED FROM:

44 physical symptoms
 8 mental symptoms   -- medical symptoms
 4 behavioural symptoms
 4 social symptoms   -- social symptoms   Mean referral
                                                            scores
   Referral gradings for all symptoms
   1 = No referral
   2 = Lay or informal referral
   3 = Professional or formal referral
                                                         Incongruous
   Medical symptom gradings for: referral scores
   pain, disability, perceived
   seriousness, duration

   Social symptom gradings for:
   worry or inconvenience

FIGURE 1.4   Dependent variables

symptoms for the purposes of calculating referral scores. Each
subject therefore had three pairs of referral scores. The first
pair measured the tendency of an individual to refer medical and
social symptoms formally. These were the mean referral scores
calculated from the referral gradings of 1 for no referral, 2 for
an informal referral, and 3 for a formal referral, and allowing for
the different numbers of symptoms per person. The minority of
subjects with no symptoms could not have referral scores.

The second pair of referral scores defined and identified those
who were part of the symptom 'iceberg' for medical and social
symptoms. These were people who did not refer symptoms for professional advice although they themselves considered that the pain
or disability was severe (or worry for social symptoms) or that the
symptom was serious. These were not therefore value-judgments made
by some observer about what people should or should not do, but
calculations based entirely upon an individual's subjective perception of their own symptoms.

The converse of the symptom 'iceberg' was symptom 'trivia',
which implies that symptoms were taken unnecessarily for professional
advice. Again it was the subject's own evaluation of their symptoms
that was used as the basis of definition rather than someone else's
opinion about appropriateness. People with 'trivia' were those who
sought professional advice about symptoms which they themselves
said caused no pain or disability (or only slight worry for social
symptoms), and which they did not think were serious. These four
incongruous referral scores therefore operationalized the concepts
of the symptom 'iceberg' and 'trivia', which until now have tended
to be vague value-judgments, usually reflecting the point of view
of those who make them, rather than any rational appraisal of
people's behaviour.

As well as defining referral behaviour, the scores for referral
and symptom prevalence related to subjects rather than to discrete
symptoms, and could therefore be correlated with other attributes of
individuals such as the sociographic data. These are the independent variables which fall into broad categories as indicated in
Figure 1.5. The stages of the analysis are shown diagrammatically
in Figure 1.6, and represent different levels of conceptualization.
It may be misleading to make deductions between correlations at one
level with those of another.(36)

The basis of the study was descriptive data about the perception
and referral of symptoms as presented in Chapters 3 and 4, together
with sociographic data about the subjects as described in Chapter 2,
and information about their use and perception of services in
Chapters 5 and 6. The initial data on symptoms and referral were
based on discrete symptoms rather than individual subjects, each of
whom may have had several different symptoms. In order to relate
this basic symptom data to the sociographic variables for each
subject, it was necessary to calculate composite measures of symptom
prevalence and referral behaviour for individual subjects, rather
than for each of their symptoms. These were the dependent variables
defined in Figure 1.4 and described in Chapters 3 and 4.

Associations between the dependent variables for symptom prevalence and referral behaviour, and the independent sociographic vari
ables are then described in Chapter 7 and 8, first using bivariate

Introductory:
Practice, month.

Sociographic:
Age, sex, age-sex group*, marital status, employment status, social
class, education, religion.

Housing:
Housing tenure, period when house built, type of house, number of
rooms, number of occupants, density*, toilet facilities, hot water
and fixed bath or shower, amenities*.

Mobility:
Years in present residence, years with present GP, previous residence, mother's residence at time of birth, main place of upbringing,
birth and upbringing*, number of moves, relatives seen in past week.

Past Medical History:
Past medical history, number of short hospital stays, number of long
hospital stays.

Present Health:
Self-estimate of present health, present illnesses or disabilities.

Smoking:
Smoking habits, smoking history, number of cigarettes per day,
smoking score*.

Interviewee:
Interviewee relationship, age of interviewee, sex of interviewee.

Personality and Intelligence:
Personality-extroversion, personality-neuroticism, intelligence,
medical knowledge score.

Use of Medical Services:
Visits to surgery in past year, home visits by GP in past year, how
doctor contacted, travel to health centre, minutes to health centre,
travel-time to health centre*.

Perception of Medical Services:
Experience of doctors and hospitals, preference for health centre,
suggested improvements, difficulty in contacting doctor, action on
symptom if in doubt, home remedies, which doctor preferred to see
first.

Medicine Taking:
Prescribed medicine taking, number of prescribed medicines taken,
unprescribed medicine taking, number of unprescribed medicines taken.

Use of Social Work:
Social worker seen in past year, why social worker seen.

Perception of Social Work:
Problems social worker deals with, anyone else to social worker -
who? anyone else to social worker - why? how to contact social
worker, where is nearest social work department.

Other sources of Assistance:
Other helping agencies - which? other helping agencies - why?
neighbourhood advice.

<u>Family Planning</u>:
Method of contraception, contraceptive advice, contraceptive
supplies, adequacy of contraceptive facilities.

<u>Interviewer Assessment</u>:
Condition of home, social adjustment of subject, cooperation of
interviewee, reliability of answers.

<u>Miscellaneous</u>:
Other personal matters, subject's comments on interview, length of
interview, others present during interview.

<u>Mean Grading Scales</u>:
Mean pain score*, mean disability score*, mean seriousness score*,
mean duration score*, mean worry score*.

* Computed variables.

FIGURE 1.5   Independent variables

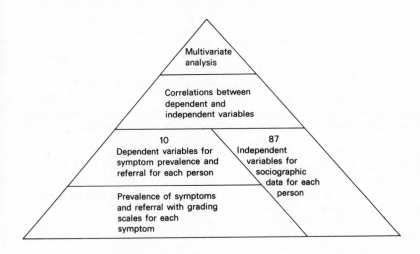

FIGURE 1.6   Diagram of analysis

and second multivariate analysis. Finally, the implications of the
findings are discussed in Chapter 9 and the conclusions summarized
in Chapter 10. Significant associations between variables are not
necessarily causal, and indicate relevant questions rather than
definite answers. It would be possible to formulate every statistical association in the form of a discrete hypothesis, but it is
more helpful to view such associations as part of a descriptive
process which can be likened to a pyramid as shown in Figure 1.6.
Multivariate analysis forms the peak of the pyramid where the
strands can be drawn together. This provides a perspective which
throws some light on a complex situation, and points the way towards
a more rational approach in the future.

REFERENCES

1 Last, J.M. (1963), The Illness Iceberg, 'Lancet', 6 July, 28-31.
2 Butler, J.R. (1970), Illness and the Sick Role; an Evaluation
   of Three Communities, 'British Journal of Sociology', 21/3,
   241-61.
3 Pearse, I.H. and Crocker, L.H. (1943), 'The Peckham Experiment',
   Allen & Unwin, London.
4 Wadsworth, M.E.J., Butterfield, W.J.H., and Blaney, R. (1971),
   'Health and Sickness: The Choice of Treatment', Tavistock,
   London.
5 Cartwright, A. (1967), 'Patients and Their Doctors: A Study of
   General Practice', Routledge & Kegan Paul, London.
6 Parsons, T. (1951), 'The Social System', Routledge & Kegan Paul,
   London.
7 Bloom, S. (1963), 'The Doctor and His Patient', Russell Sage
   Foundation, New York.
8 'Social Work (Scotland) Act' (1968), HMSO, Edinburgh.
9 Jefferys, M. (1965), 'An Anatomy of Social Welfare Services',
   Michael Joseph, London.
10 Holtermann, S. (1975), 'Census Indicators of Urban Deprivation',
   Working Note No.6, Department of the Environment, London.
11 Registrar General Scotland (1974), 'Annual Report - Part 1 -
   Mortality Statistics', HMSO, Edinburgh.
12 Dubos, R. (1965), 'Man Adapting', Yale University Press, New
   Haven and London.
13 Butterfield, W.J.H. (1968), 'Priorities in Medical Care',
   Nuffield Provincial Hospitals Trust, London.
14 Cochrane, A.L. and Fletcher, C.M. (1968), 'The Early Diagnosis
   of Some Diseases of the Lung', Office of Health Economics,
   London.
15 Rose, G.A. (1962), The Diagnosis of Ischaemic Heart Pain and
   Intermittent Claudication in Field Surveys, 'Bulletin of the
   World Health Organisation', 27, 645-58.
16 Foulds, G.A. and Hope, K. (1968), 'Manual of the Symptom-Sign
   Inventory', University of London Press.
17 Stone, F.H. (1971), Personal communication.
18 Maddox, E.J. (1971), Analysis of some data from the Drumchapel
   Family Centre, Unpublished paper.
19 HMSO (1970), 'Classification of Occupations'.
20 British Sociological Association and Social Science Research
   Council (1969), 'Comparability in Social Science', Heineman,
   London.
21 Scottish Development Department (1969), 'The New Scottish
   Housing Handbook, Bulletin 2', HMSO, Edinburgh.
22 Eysenck, H.J. (1958), A Short Questionnaire for the Measurement
   of Two Dimensions of Personality, 'Journal of Applied Psychology',
   42/1, 14-17.
23 Gilmore, A.J.J. (1972), Personality in the Elderly: Problems in
   Methodology, 'Age and Ageing', 1, 227.
24 Cattell, R.B., Eber, H.W., and Tatsuoka, M.M. (1970), 'Handbook
   for the 16 Personality Factor (Form C-1963)', Institute for
   Personality and Ability Testing, USA.

25   Richardson, I.M. and Dingwall-Fordyce, I. (1968), Patient
     Geography in General Practice, 'Lancet', 7581, 1290-3.
26   Gilmore, A.J.J. and Caird, F.I. (1972), Locating the Elderly
     at Home, 'Age and Ageing', 1, 30-2.
27   Moser, C.A. and Kalton, G. (1971), 'Survey Methods in Social
     Investigation', Heinemann Educational, London.
28   Hannay, D.R. (1972), The Accuracy of Health Centre Records,
     'Lancet', 19 August, 371-3.
29   Hollingsworth, T.H. (1970), 'Migration: A Study Based on
     Scottish Experience', Oliver & Boyd, Edinburgh.
30   Smith, M. (1973), Moonlight Flittings in Glasgow, 'Scotsman',
     4 May.
31   Hotson, J. (1973), Personal communication.
32   Nie, N.H., Bent, D.H., and Hull, C.H. (1970), 'Statistical
     Package for the Social Sciences', McGraw-Hill, New York.
33   Statistical Package for Social Sciences (1973), 'Update Manual',
     Edinburgh University.
34   Blalock, M.M. (1972), 'Social Statistics', McGraw-Hill
     Kogakusha, Tokyo.
35   Documenta Geigy (1970), 'Scientific Tables', J.R. Geigy,
     Switzerland.
36   Susser, M. (1973), 'Causal Thinking in the Health Sciences',
     Oxford University Press.

Chapter 2

THE PEOPLE

'Then gently scan your brother man
Still gentler sister woman.'

(Robert Burns 1759-96)

Both symptoms and referral behaviour depend on the people being studied and the environment in which they live. It is therefore important that the context in which the research was carried out should be adequately described in terms of the subjects involved and their physical and social background. In this way the relevance of the findings can be brought into focus, not only for a particular place and time, but in the wider context of the urban environment of modern man.

PERSONAL ATTRIBUTES

The age-sex distribution of those interviewed is shown in Figure 2.1, and indicates that they were almost equally divided between males (47 per cent) and females (53 per cent). When compared by five-year age-groups, the survey sample closely reflected the population of both Glasgow (1) and Scotland,(2) with 28 per cent under 15 years old and almost 13 per cent over 65. The main difference was that those in their thirties tended to be under-represented in the survey, probably because their greater mobility and health made them more likely to be amongst the non-responders as already described. Almost all those who answered for children were parents, mostly mothers, and over half were in their thirties. Of the 5 per cent who were not parents the largest group were grandparents, followed by elder siblings.

The personality and intelligence tests were self-completed by all respondents whether answering for themselves or children. Of those interviewed 8 per cent did not do the personality tests and 14 per cent did not do the intelligence test, although both were very short - the former having twelve questions and the latter eight. A few elderly people were too blind or deaf to do the tests, but at least some of these refusals were due to adult illiteracy, while others said they did not understand the questions. The

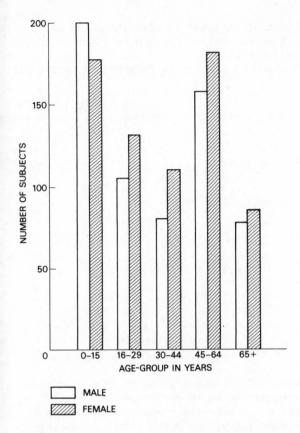

FIGURE 2.1 Age-sex distribution of sample

personality test gave two scores for extroversion and neuroticism
between 0 and 6. The mean score for those interviewed was 3.5 for
extroversion and 2.8 for neuroticism. These compared with 4.0 and
3.1 respectively for the original test means,(3) although the
questions had been slightly modified. Very few people achieved a
high score on the intelligence test, for which the mean score was
2.5, compared to an adult norm of 3.8 given for this particular
test.(4)

SOCIAL CHARACTERISTICS

The marital status of those interviewed reflected the proportions
in the City of Glasgow (1) with 46 per cent being single, 43 per
cent married, and 8 per cent widows or widowers. However, 3 per
cent of the sample said they were separated or divorced, which is
about three times the number given in the 1971 census for divorcees
in Glasgow. The difference probably represents the large number of
broken marriages in which couples were separated without being
legally divorced.
     Just over 10 per cent of subjects were unemployed, and less than
half of these because of illness. This figure is higher than the

8 per cent given for West Central Scotland in 1972,(5) which in
turn was more than the Scottish and United Kingdom averages of 6
and 4 per cent respectively for that year.
     The social class distribution of the sample is shown in Figure 2.2.

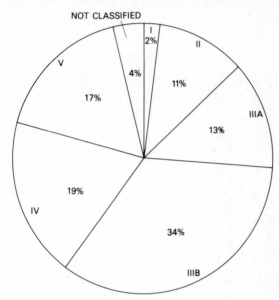

FIGURE 2.2 Social class
distribution of
sample (1,344 subjects)

This classification is a very crude ranking scale based on occupation, which has tended to be superseded by socio-economic groups
for population data in Britain. A comparison with the 1966 sample
census (6) showed that the survey subjects were broadly representative of the social class composition of the country, except that
there was twice the percentage of social class V amongst those
interviewed, with corresponding small reductions for all the other
social classes.
     Education was assessed by length of full-time formal education.
Only 12 per cent had had any full-time further education, the
remaining 60 per cent of adults having left school at ages ranging
between 13 and 15, depending on the school leaving age at the time.
     A distinction was made between active and passive religious
affiliation, because for many people their religion or denomination
is purely nominal. Overall, 41 per cent had an active religious
affiliation and 55 per cent were only passive, with the remaining
4 per cent being unclassified. The categories are shown in Figure
2.3, which indicates striking differences in the proportions of those
who were active participants, with 71 per cent for non-Christians,
59 per cent for Roman Catholics, 43 per cent for other Protestant
denominations, and only 31 per cent for the Church of Scotland. The
first group were likely to be recent immigrants from the Indian sub-
continent, the second group mainly of Irish extraction, and the
third group from elsewhere in the United Kingdom. One explanation
of these differences might be that distance from a cultural base
increases religious allegiance as a focus of stability for minority
groups. Conversely, an indigenous urban population might be less
likely to express its identity through religious observance.

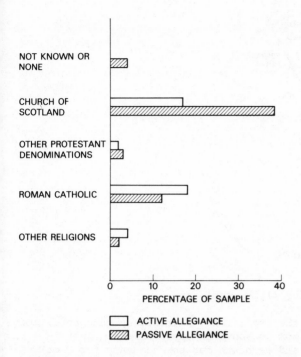

FIGURE 2.3 Religious allegiance (1,344 subjects)

Although 30 per cent of those interviewed had not seen any
relative in the previous week, the majority had fairly frequent
contacts, which occurred at least daily for over 20 per cent of
subjects, apart from members of their own household.

HOUSING

Of those interviewed 46 per cent were corporation tenants, and only
23 per cent were owner-occupiers. Of the remainder, many were
tenants of the Scottish Special Housing Association, as well as
renting from private landlords. Housing in Scotland, and particularly in Glasgow, is dominated by local authority tenancies, which
are more than double the proportion of those in England and Wales.
(7) Conversely, only about 25 per cent of people are owner-
occupiers in Scotland, which is half the percentage elsewhere in
the United Kingdom.

About 44 per cent of subjects lived in housing built before the
First World War, mostly in traditional stone-built tenements of four
storeys; 26 per cent of the houses in the survey were built between
the two world wars, many in large peripheral housing estates. The
remaining 30 per cent of dwellings were post-1944, and often high
rise blocks of flats.

The types of dwelling found in the survey are shown in Figure
2.4. Only 15 per cent lived in houses with their own front door to
the street, and 11 per cent lived in post-war high rise flats. A
distinction was made between the lower four floors of high flats,

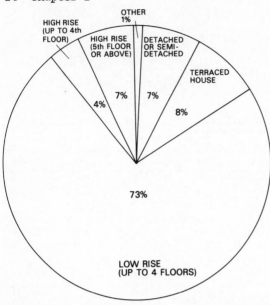

FIGURE 2.4   Type of housing (1,344 subjects)

which were equivalent to the traditional four-storey tenements, and
dwellings on the fifth floor or above of tower blocks.   Again
Glasgow both accentuates and accounts for the tendency for Scotland
to have more flat-dwellers (43 per cent of households) than England
and Wales (17 per cent of households).(7)

The commonest size of dwelling was a three-roomed apartment
which comprised 43 per cent of the sample, with about 20 per cent
each having either two or four rooms; 3 per cent of dwellings were
single rooms, and the remaining 14 per cent had five or more rooms.
If anything single room accommodation in Glasgow was under-
represented in the survey.(8)   The numbers of occupants normally
resident in the houses visited were very similar to figures for
Glasgow as a whole,(1) with two-thirds being about equally divided
between households of two, three, four, or five persons.   At the
ends of the scale, 8 per cent of those interviewed lived alone, and
almost one-quarter were in dwellings with six or more in the home.
The size of households in terms of numbers of occupants and rooms,
was combined to give a density of persons per room.   Over half those
interviewed lived at a density of more than one person per room,
which is similar to figures for Glasgow (1) but a much higher proportion than for Scotland as a whole (17 per cent) or England and Wales
(5 per cent).(7)   Almost one in five subjects were living with two
or more people per room, and there were eight respondents with a
density of four or more per room.

The great majority of dwellings had their own inside toilet, but
almost 10 per cent did not, most of these having a shared outside
toilet on the tenement stairs.   Over three-quarters had both hot
water and a fixed bath or shower, but almost 15 per cent of homes
had neither.   The presence or absence of an inside toilet, hot water,
and a fixed bath or shower, were combined into a single variable for
basic amenities.   Three-quarters of the households in the survey had
all three amenities, but there were a hundred subjects who had no

amenities apart from an outside toilet, and three did not even have that. Again these findings reflected the situation in Glasgow as a whole.(1)

One of the assessments made by the interviewers was the condition of the home, because this often bore little relation to the external appearances of a building or to the presence of basic amenities. Even the most derelict tenements often contained well-kept homes once inside the front door, whereas some flats in well-built areas with every amenity were in a very bad state with little furniture or attempt at housekeeping. About 10 per cent of homes were graded as poor, reflecting the sometimes appalling conditions in which some subjects lived. However, 43 per cent were rated as good, and the remainder were average or unspecified.

The circumstances in which many subjects lived reflected the extent of the housing problem in Scotland, where it was estimated there were over a quarter of a million unfit homes.(9) The bulk of the problem lay in Glasgow, where almost a quarter of the housing was considered to be below a tolerable standard in 1970.(5) As a result there has been an extensive programme of slum clearance, which has left whole areas of the city demolished or derelict. Unfortunately, houses were condemned long before demolition or replacement took place, and the subsequent 'planning blight' de-graded the environment in which so many Glasgow families lived. During the year the survey was being carried out, over 6,500 houses were closed or demolished while less than 400 were designated for improvement; and during this period over 20,000 houses were standing empty, or 7 per cent of the total housing stock of the city.(8) To add to these difficulties, rehousing policies have created new problems such as the dereliction of inter-war council houses from lack of upkeep,(10) and the effects of high flats, especially on families with young children.(11)

The situations in which families often found themselves when living in slum clearance areas can best be illustrated by the follow-ing interviewer's comments:

9-year-old girl: 'Family living in appalling conditions. Most of property demolished. Back court overrun by rats. House very dirty.'

36-year-old wife of unemployed plasterer: 'The main reason for wanting to move was to get away from the area because of vandalism due to all the demolitions in the streets round about.'

40-year-old divorced housewife: 'Tenements on either side near-derelict; she is on top landing, floor below empty. Afraid to go out shopping, barricades door at night. Fear has also infected daughter.'

1-year-old daughter of a bus conductor: 'Daughter's main trouble was head-lice. Family of four in one room. Walls damp. Ground floor of building derelict. Condemned, family waiting to be re-housed - but only offered slum in rough area, so refused.'

8-year-old daughter of a lorry driver: 'Parents and five children on top floor of half-derelict tenement. Roof leaked; drain in close

overflowing.   Child reluctant to go out to play; had to be pushed
out - no other children in close.   Other nearby properties derelict.'

Clearly such comments refer only to a minority, but the fact remains
that the Clydeside area of Scotland has by far the highest concentration of urban deprivation in the United Kingdom, as measured by
such as census indicators as overcrowding, lack of basic amenities,
and unemployment.(12)   Unfortunately, the way in which slum clearance has been carried out has tended to increase the difficulties
of families living in such areas (13,14) with problems of vandalism
following in the wake of dereliction.

MOBILITY

The extent of mobility in the Glasgow conurbation had already been
mentioned in relation to the survey response rate.   Extensive
redevelopment increases the amount of internal mobility as families
are rehoused, often in overspill housing schemes, so that the population of the central city had steadily declined.(1)   The average
length of stay for subjects at their present address was about
seven-and-a-half years.   This was almost certainly an over-estimate
for the population in general, because the more frequent movers
were less likely to be at the address given for them.   Nevertheless,
the average length of registration with a doctor was almost double
this at just over fourteen years, reflecting the tendency for
patients to remain with their family doctor although they themselves
were moving within the conurbation.   These two variables of length
of residence at one address, and length of registration with a
doctor, are compared in Figure 2.5.

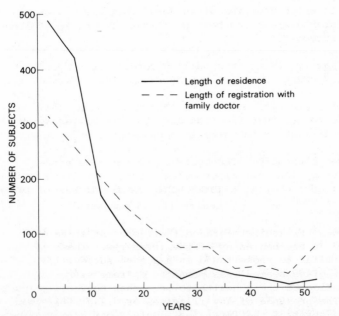

FIGURE 2.5   Length of residence and registration with family doctor

Less than 10 per cent of those interviewed had moved to their
present address from outside Glasgow, and over three-quarters had
been born and brought up in the city. Of the remainder about 9 per
cent had been born and brought up elsewhere in Scotland, 4 per cent
had come from England, Wales or Ireland, and another 4 per cent were
from overseas. These latter were mainly immigrants from India and
Pakistan, who were over-represented in the survey,(1) because they
tended to congregate in older housing in the central area served by
the health centre. Most had come as adults and many spoke little
English, especially the wives.

The average number of changes of address for those interviewed
was three, which was almost certainly an under-estimate for the
population as a whole because of the response bias. About 18 per
cent of subjects had moved five or more times, and ten people had
had over fourteen moves.

PAST AND PRESENT HEALTH

In reply to initial questions on past and present health over 40 per
cent of subjects said that they had had no serious illness, accidents or operations in the past, excluding minor ailments, childhood
infections and childbirth. As many as 30 per cent had never been
an inpatient in hospital and less than 5 per cent had been a long-
stay patient for six months or more.

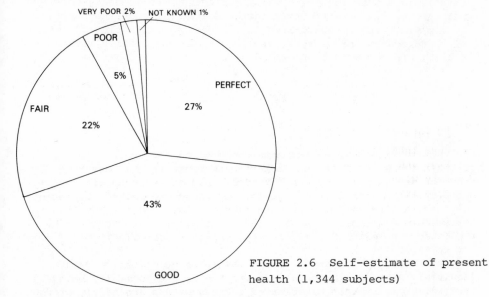

FIGURE 2.6   Self-estimate of present
health (1,344 subjects)

Figure 2.6 shows how subjects graded their present state of
health when asked at the beginning of the interview. These self-
estimates were similar to those found in a London survey,(15)
except that Glaswegians seemed less prone to extreme statements
in that fewer considered their health to be either perfect, or poor
and very poor. The presence of any illnesses or disabilities was
also asked at the start of the interview. Only 2 per cent mentioned

more than two illnesses or disabilities, and 64 per cent said they had none. This compares reasonably with the 70 per cent who thought their health was good or perfect, but was very much more than the 14 per cent who were subsequently found to be symptomless on detailed questioning. These findings raise doubts about the value of health indices based on very general questions.(16,17)

Details of cigarette smoking were asked in view of its importance as a cause of ill-health,(18) and because Glasgow has some of the highest known rates for diseases such as lung-cancer, together with a high consumption of cigarettes.(19) Questions were asked only of adults about the number of cigarettes smoked, whether they inhaled, and whether they had given up smoking and if so when. The results were combined for the purposes of analysis into a single smoking score as shown in Figure 2.7. This indicates that over half the

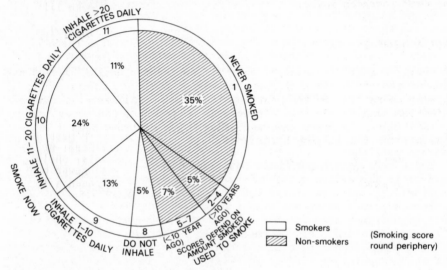

FIGURE 2.7 Smoking habits (964 adults)

adults interviewed were cigarette smokers and the great majority of these inhaled. Most non-smokers were those who had never started, and only 12 per cent of adults had given up smoking - the majority within the last ten years. Of those who smoked at present only one in five smoked more than twenty a day, and few admitted to heavy chain-smoking. These figures are similar to those given by the Tobacco Research Council for the United Kingdom.(20)

The brief description above, based mainly on quantitative data, inevitably gives an inadequate impression of the community being studied. Some aspects are blurred whereas others are barely brought into focus. For instance, there were no specific questions about alcohol consumption, because answers to this tend to be unreliable and were anyhow intended to come under social symptoms. In the event it did not figure prominently in the results, partly because of reticence, and partly because one person's alcohol problem may be another man's social drinking, especially in the context of Glasgow's norms of behaviour.

Another over-riding impression of the area being studied was the speed of change. People were continually moving as 'planning blight' spread like a disease to whole neighbourhoods. Some old tenements, however, were still part of thriving local communities, whilst other more recent council housing was bleak in the extreme, especially in the peripheral estates built between the wars, with few shops or community centres. There was little attempt at landscaping round the new high-rise flats, where people seemed bewildered by a vertical anonymity, which unreliable lifts did little to alleviate. Addresses were impersonal numbers, and entrance notices forbidding loitering or ball games mingled with graffiti to add to the atmosphere of anomie.

There were several indications that the less articulate, and especially the elderly living on their own, missed out on the social services available. Often they became isolated as families moved away and neighbourhoods disintegrated with redevelopment. One 55-year-old respondent said that she would like to have it known that she was most concerned about the lack of attention to old people.

But it would be a mistake to leave an impression of unrelieved gloom. The great majority of respondents were friendly and helpful, and most welcomed the chance of talking about themselves. Some housing areas were admirable, and Glasgow's parks, like the surrounding countryside, are both accessible and beautiful. The location and potential are there for a satisfying and fulfilling urban environment, but this would require above all a change of public and private attitudes.

There were many happy homes but also a great deal of distress, much of it associated with the environment, and particularly with housing, irrespective of the age of buildings. One respondent expressed doubts about the wisdom of collecting health facts when the overwhelming need was for new housing. However, the quality of life did not depend only on the newness of houses, but also on the attitudes and stability of the inhabitants. In some areas with all the basic amenities, streets were littered with broken glass, and mongrels roamed in packs, being owned apparently more for protection than as pets. Some parents seemed to have lost control and schools were unable to cope, as children slipped down the slopes of truancy, vandalism and crime. On the other hand, many families were being happily brought up in less than ideal conditions. If there were any heroes of this story it would be the many mothers who created comfortable and cheerful homes, in spite of their physical and social environment, as illustrated by the following interviewer's comment: 'A good caring family who had made a decent home on the top floor of an appalling crumbling tenement, which is due for demolition.'

Although these comments relate to one particular city with perhaps more than its share of difficulties, these are common throughout the Western world. Industrial society has created an urban environment where deprivation and renewal may combine with social and family instability. The resulting community problems are too complex for individuals to remedy and administrative structures are often inappropriate. It is against this background that the health of modern man is determined.

REFERENCES

1   Registrar General Scotland (1973), 'County Report: City of
    Glasgow Census 1971, Scotland', HMSO, Edinburgh.
2   Registrar General Scotland (1973), 'Annual Report 1972, Part 1',
    HMSO, Edinburgh.
3   Eysenck, H.J. (1969), 'Manual of the Maudsley Personality
    Inventory', University of London Press.
4   Kear-Colwell, J.J. (1973), Personal communication.
5   Buchanan, C. et al. (1974), 'West Central Scotland - A pro-
    gramme of action', Consultative draft report, Glasgow.
6   Central Statistical Office (1973), 'Social Trends No.4', HMSO,
    London.
7   Office of Population Censuses and Surveys (1973), 'The General
    Household Survey', HMSO, London.
8   Corporation of the City of Glasgow (1972), 'Report of the
    Medical Officer of Health', Glasgow.
9   Scottish Housing Advisory Committee (1967), 'Scotland's Older
    Housing', Scottish Development Department, Edinburgh.
10 Scottish Housing Advisory Committee (1970), 'Council House
    Communities', Scottish Development Department, Edinburgh.
11 Jephcott, P. (1971), 'Homes in High Flats', Oliver & Boyd,
    Edinburgh.
12 Holtermann, S. (1975), 'Census Indicators of Urban Deprivation',
    Working Note No.6, Department of the Environment, London.
13 English, J. and Norman, P. (1974), 'One Hundred Years of Slum
    Clearance in England and Wales - Policies and Programmes
    1868-1970', Discussion Papers in Social Research No.1, University
    of Glasgow.
14 English, J. and Norman, P. (1974), 'An Appraisal of Slum Clear-
    ance Procedures in England and Wales', Discussion Papers in
    Social Research No.4, University of Glasgow.
15 Office of Health Economics (1968), 'Without Prescription',
    London.
16 Grogono, A.W. and Woodgate, D.J. (1971), Index for Measuring
    Health, 'Lancet', 7732, 1024-6.
17 'Lancet' (1973), Measuring Health and Disease, 7815, 1293-4.
18 Royal College of Physicians (1971), 'Smoking and Health Now',
    Pitman Medical, London.
19 Haddow, A.J. (1967), 'Annual Report', Western Regional Cancer
    Registration Bureau, Glasgow.
20 Todd, G.F. (1972), 'Statistics of Smoking in the United Kingdom',
    Tobacco Research Council, London.

Chapter 3

PREVALENCE OF SYMPTOMS

'That man yet never knew
The way to health that durst not show his sore.'
          Francis Beaumont (1584-1616) and John Fletcher (1579-1625)

The questions on specific symptoms were asked in a grouped form so
that two or three related symptoms were asked together, as shown in
Appendix I. The prevalence of symptoms is described below for each
of the main types of symptoms - namely physical, mental, behavioural,
and social. The findings for the symptom grading scales are then
given, and finally the results of the computed scores for the
frequency per person of the four main types of symptoms.

PHYSICAL SYMPTOMS

A detailed breakdown of the results for each symptom question is
given in Appendix II. This shows the two-week period prevalence
for each individual symptom, as well as for the forty-four symptom
groups, expressed as a percentage of the total sample interviewed.
Looking first at the groups of symptoms, respiratory symptoms were
by far the commonest, followed by headaches, and feeling tired or
generally run down. Trouble with the feet, ears, eyes and skin came
next, together with varicose veins and cardio-respiratory symptoms
such as shortness of breath and ankle swelling. When these groups
are broken down into individual symptoms, those with a prevalence of
more than 10 per cent are shown in Figure 3.1. Where an individual
symptom occurred in combination, this has been added to the prevalence for the single symptom. Again there was a striking preponderance of respiratory symptoms together with those of general malaise
such as tiredness and headaches. Apart from these, trouble with
the feet, skin, varicose veins, and hearing were the commonest
individual symptoms.
    It is possible to gain some idea of broader medical categories
by combining groups of symptoms, as shown in Figure 3.2. This
involves assumptions about cause which may be arbitrary (e.g.
placing 'shortness of breath' with the respiratory rather than

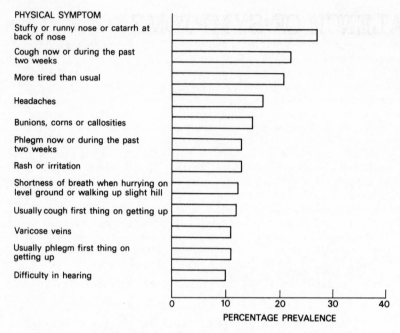

FIGURE 3.1   Commonest physical symptoms (1,344 subjects)

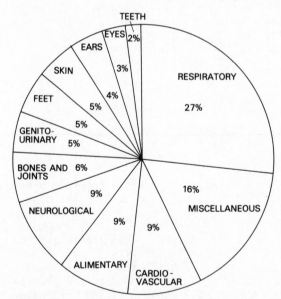

FIGURE 3.2   Physical symptom categories (5,737 symptoms for all
             subjects)

cardiovascular system), and the retention of original symptom
groupings which might have been split between symptoms (e.g. leaving
'difficulty with swallowing' with teeth rather than the alimentary
system).   Inevitably there is also a large miscellaneous category.
      The questions on physical symptoms were asked of all 1,344 adults

and children, and were phrased in simple lay language. Nevertheless, several such symptoms can be translated into medical terminology with varying degrees of diagnostic implication. For instance from the questions on chronic cough and phlegm it seemed that about 12 per cent of all those studied had chronic bronchitis, and at least 49 people had symptoms suggestive of asthma. There were also two cases of haemoptysis. The questions on shortness of breath were worded according to grades of dyspnoea, for which 260 subjects had varying degrees and 30 had paroxysmal nocturnal dyspnoea.

Questions on the cardiovascular system indicated 26 people with angina, 18 with the symptoms of coronary thrombosis, and a further 51 with ill-defined pain or discomfort in the chest, which is a much commoner symptom than is usually recognized medically.(1) There were 17 people with intermittent claudication, 81 with leg cramps (mainly nocturnal), and 125 with varicose veins.

Questions on the locomotor and nervous systems suggested there may have been 29 cases of rheumatoid arthritis, and 5 of epilepsy. Less specifically, there were 72 people with low back pain, 16 with ataxia, and 6 with aphasia. There were 130 subjects with some degree of motor or sensory loss in their limbs, and 20 who were blind in one or both eyes.

Although some conditions such as angina and chronic bronchitis are defined in terms of symptoms, it is not possible in a subjective study to be certain about those diagnoses which are not so defined, but for which single symptoms are highly suggestive. For instance, 75 people had urinary frequency and 16 dysuria, and there were 3 cases of possible jaundice. It is likely that the woman with bleeding in pregnancy had a threatened miscarriage, but less so that those who felt 'more thirsty than usual' had diabetes.

It is difficult to compare the results of this study with others because of the conceptual confusions which underlie surveys into health and illness, such as failure to distinguish between symptoms and diagnoses.(2) There have been many morbidity surveys purporting to measure ill health in the community. Some have used subjective scales and scores without being explicit about symptoms.(3) Others have defined ill health in terms of both symptoms such as chest pains, and chronic conditions such as asthma or piles which are really diagnoses.(4,5) At the other extreme are morbidity surveys which depend on physical examination.(6)

Pearse and Crocker (7) distinguished between 'dis-eases' which people felt subjectively, and 'dis-orders' which were discovered objectively on examination. There might be no physical cause found for a 'dis-ease' and 'dis-orders' might be presymptomatic if found on screening. This precise semantic distinction has not gained currency and the best medical equivalents today are symptoms and signs. Symptoms are by definition subjective whereas signs are objective. They are quite distinct concepts with the exception of self-perceived signs such as painless bleeding or lumps, which people notice about themselves through the medium of their five senses. Symptoms do not necessarily imply ill health or disease; one can be tired or breathless without being ill. Symptoms may be classified in many different ways,(8) and the diagnoses given by doctors even to common symptoms may vary widely.(9) In addition the interpretation of common medical terms may be very different for doctors and patients.(10)

To the problems of definition and communication are added those
of reliability and validity. One study (11) found that item specif-
icity as attempted in this survey increased reliability, but concluded that validity depended on the original intent. If the intent
was to record subjective symptoms as in the present study, then there
is no objective way of verifying such data. If, however, the intent
was to measure ill health, then the validity of reported symptoms
could be tested by physical examination as a measure of ill health,
depending on the definitions used. Several studies have looked at
the validity of measures of ill health,(12) either for questionnaires
(13) or household interviews.(14) Survey data on the physical
health of residents in California were checked against medical
records for validity, and by repeat interviews for reliability;(15)
it was found that only 54 per cent of chronic conditions reported
on the survey were present on the clinical records, but that responses for these conditions were 96 per cent reliable. Other studies
from America have found that mothers were likely to over-report
aspects of family health,(16) and that reinforcement produced a 25
per cent increase in health items reported at interview.(17) But
these investigations tended to define health in terms of diagnoses
rather than subjective symptoms, which in a sense are only valid for
one person, and only reliable at one time.

In spite of differences in methodology the predominance of
respiratory symptoms has been confirmed in other community studies
in the United Kingdom,(4,5) Australia,(18) and America.(19)
Although it is important to distinguish between such surveys and
those based on reported morbidity in general practice, these latter
studies have also found that respiratory conditions were the commonest diagnoses.(20,21) Reported morbidity is also different from
mortality, but it has been estimated that 14 per cent of all deaths
in Scotland are due to respiratory disease.(22)

A standard method for recording symptoms of ischaemic heart pain
and intermittent claudication has been developed,(23) and was used
in this survey, although even these questions have been found to be
subject to response variation.(24) In the present study, 9 per
cent of all physical symptoms were classified as relating to the
cardiovascular system, which was very similar to findings from
Australia,(18) Germany (25) and Norway,(26) although the methods
used were not always comparable. Two recent surveys in the United
Kingdom (4,5) did not seem to have employed any accepted methodology
for recording cardiovascular symptoms.

In the present study, 9 per cent of all physical symptoms were
classified as alimentary and the same proportion as neurological.
These figures are similar to those from general practice in Scotland
(27) and Norway,(26) and from community surveys in England.(4) Of
physical symptoms in the present study 6 per cent related to bones
and joints, and 5 per cent to the genito-urinary system. The former
proportion is similar to findings from general practice in Scotland,
(27) but less than community surveys in England (4) or Australia,(18)
probably reflecting problems of definition rather than real differences in morbidity.(28) The amount of genito-urinary symptoms found
in Glasgow appeared to be more than double those found in London,(4)
but again differences in classification make comparisons difficult.
The same is true for skin conditions,(29) although if allowances are

made for the way in which symptoms were grouped, such as those relating to feet, the prevalence of skin complaints found in the present study appears similar to those from other surveys in the United Kingdom.(4,5)

The relationship between symptoms, diagnoses and ill health is complex and involves problems of definition which are not resolved by semantic devices such as using the word 'complaints'. For instance, the symptoms of iron-deficiency anaemia have been found to be unrelated to haemoglobin levels except for pallor in women, (30) and even this was a poor guide.(31)   Indeed the symptoms often associated with anaemia such as fatigue and headaches seem more related to neuroticism scores than the composition of the blood, (32) and in one study a quarter of those with headaches were considered to be suffering from a depressive illness.(33)   In the present study 23 per cent of those interviewed felt more tired or run-down than usual, 17 per cent said they had had headaches during the previous two weeks, and 1 per cent thought they were paler than usual.   It is difficult to draw any conclusions about ill health from such findings, and still less to make diagnostic inferences.

MENTAL SYMPTOMS

The questions on mental symptoms were asked of adults only, and as for physical symptoms, referred to the previous two weeks only.   The detailed results for each question are given in Appendix II.   These questions were derived from a Symptom Sign Inventory (34) and arranged in eight groups, the prevalence of which is also indicated in Appendix II, expressed as a percentage of all adults.   The questions were phrased in simple language without the use of medical or diagnostic terms.   None of the questions were very specific and those which correlated highly with a particular diagnosis were also likely to be positive for other psychiatric conditions.   Positive responses, therefore, tended to cluster together and indicated general psychiatric morbidity rather than specific diagnoses.

Nevertheless, it was possible to group the questions into diagnostic categories which are shown in Figure 3.3.   Where individual symptoms also occurred in combinations these have been added to the number for the single question, and the whole expressed as a percentage of the total number of mental symptoms.   All the questions fell into one of the original diagnostic categories from the Symptom Sign Inventory (34) except for the question on loneliness, which seemed an important subjective response without itself implying a psychiatric condition.

About a fifth of the adults interviewed exhibited symptoms which suggested an anxiety state and/or depression, with psychotic (or endogenous) depression predominating over neurotic (or reactive) depression.   It is not possible to arrive at a precise diagnostic prevalence because any subject with a positive response was likely to have had other mental symptoms which were not specific for particular diagnoses.   In addition, the number of mental symptoms found depended partly on the number asked.

None of the psychiatric diagnoses were mutually exclusive, and the preponderance of symptoms relating to anxiety and depression may

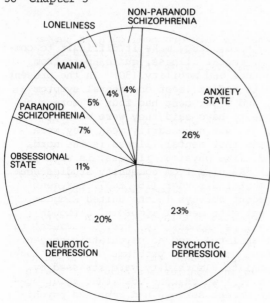

FIGURE 3.3   Mental symptom categories (1,304 symptoms for adults)

have been due to the fact that these are frequent components of
other conditions such as schizophrenia. Anxiety is also likely to
be part of a depressive or obsessional state. None the less it was
striking that 19 per cent of all adults said they felt so low in
spirits that they sat for hours on end, 17 per cent had difficulty
in getting off to sleep without sleeping pills, and 16 per cent felt
anxious at times without knowing the reason why.

A number of psychiatric screening questionnaires have been
devised with check-lists of symptoms,(35,36,37,38) but the inventory
used had attempted to validate each question against subsequent
diagnoses. However, there are problems in validating psychiatric
questionnaires,(39) and the cultural context may be important for
both the form and content of psychiatric illness.(40) There are
also considerable variations amongst psychiatrists in defining types
of mental illness, for which the symptoms are also in a sense the
signs.

As well as the difficulties of definition and methodology there
are also more fundamental conceptual problems in assessing mental
illness, which may be considered as arising mainly from the individual or society.(41) Whereas biological norms may be relatively
easy to define, social norms are complex and subjective. Estimates
of psychiatric morbidity may vary with the theoretical orientation
of the investigator,(42) and be viewed, for instance, as an aspect
of labelling for deviant behaviour,(43) or a violation of the
informal rules for the management of personal space.(44) Patients
may perceive mental illness in terms of causation,(45) and the
public perhaps accepts mental ill health as being more normative
when causes are located in early childhood,(46) and rely on disturb-
ances in interpersonal relationships to detect and explain mental
illness.(47) However, several studies suggest that families tend
to deny mental illness,(48) and people are likely to be told to do
nothing or to pull themselves together rather than go to a psychia-
trist.(49)

Problems of methodology and terminology make it difficult to compare epidemiological studies of mental illness, quite apart from
variations in population structure and mobility.(50)   In the present
study, 51 per cent of all adults had at least one mental symptom
with a mean of one per adult, and 8 per cent had four or more such
symptoms.   However, for someone to have said they were mildly
anxious, lonely or obsessive, did not necessarily mean they were
mentally ill, unless one assumes that mental illness is the norm
rather than the exception, and, like physical illness, is with the
majority most of the time.(51)   Results from community studies seem
to vary from 8 per cent with mental disorder (18) to 77 per cent
with mild phobias.(52)   Two recent surveys in the United Kingdom,
(4,5) reported about 21 per cent with mental symptoms, although
definitions varied from 'mental, psychoneurotic, etc. disorders' to
'nerves, depression, and irritability', and no psychiatric screening
procedures appeared to have been used.   The problems of methodology
in population surveys for psychiatric morbidity were stressed by
the Central Statistical Office,(53) which concluded that about one-
third of adults interviewed in recent surveys had reported psychiatric symptoms.

There have been several studies of mental ill health presenting
to general practice, but this only represents the tip of an iceberg.
The great majority of those with mental symptoms in the present
survey did not seek professional advice.   In one study of suburban
general practice in England,(54) one-fifth of patients had conspicuous psychiatric morbidity, and half as many again had hidden
psychiatric ill health, with the latter mainly differing in their
attitude to mental illness and usually presenting with physical
symptoms.   Similar proportions of about 20 per cent of patients
presenting with conspicuous psychiatric morbidity have been
reported from rural Wales (55) and urban Sweden,(56) but progres-
sively smaller percentages from comparable studies in the Netherlands,(57) Australia,(58) and semi-rural Scotland.(27)   The diversity
of criteria used to define psychiatric morbidity makes comparisons
difficult, but there is some evidence that more psychoneurotic conditions are being referred to general practitioners.(59)

A study of psychiatric conditions seen in general practice,(60)
reported that 40 per cent had anxiety neurosis, 42 per cent neurotic
depression, and 8 per cent psychotic depression.   These are higher
proportions than from the present study except for psychotic
depression, which may be the least likely to be referred for
medical advice.   The diagnosis of depression is therefore an
important part of primary care as it is a treatable and potentially
lethal condition.(61)   Most depressions, however, include symptoms
of anxiety,(62) and where the latter predominate somatic symptoms
may increase.(63)   From the present survey, 10 per cent of positive
mental symptoms pointed towards a diagnosis of schizophrenia.
Several studies have supported the extent to which some symptoms
are characteristic of schizophrenia,(64,65) and also the way in
which symptoms distinguish between neurotic and psychotic depression.
(66,67)

BEHAVIOURAL SYMPTOMS

The questions on behavioural symptoms were asked of those answering
for children of 15 years or under, and were derived from the commonest presenting symptoms at a Department of Child Psychiatry,(68)
and from developmental milestones. The detailed results are given
in Appendix II. Apart from the first two questions, the remainder
were asked of specific age-groups only. A breakdown of the responses
by age-groups is therefore shown in Table 3.1. Almost a quarter of
the children in the survey had at least one behavioural symptom.

TABLE 3.1   Children's behavioural symptoms

| Behavioural symptom group | Number of behavioural symptoms (% for each age-group in brackets) | | | | |
| | Age-group in years | | | | Total |
	0-2	3-5	6-10	11-15	
More difficult to manage (cries, temper, disobedience)	1 (2%)	12 (16%)	15 (11%)	5 (4%)	33
More difficult to manage (in other ways)	2 (4%)	7 (9%)	9 (7%)	9 (8%)	27
Not alert or not smiling	0	-	-	-	0
Difficulty in sitting up, crawling, standing, or walking	0	-	-	-	0
Difficulty in playing with other children	-	3 (4%)	-	-	3
Difficulty with talking or sleeping	-	14 (18%)	-	-	14
Difficulty with friends or at school	-	-	17 (12%)	-	17
Bed-wetting	-	-	17 (12%)	-	17
Difficulty with friends or at school	-	-	-	13 (11%)	13
Getting into trouble	-	-	-	6 (5%)	6
Total number of behavioural symptoms	3	36	58	33	130
Number of children in each age-group	48	77	139	116	380
% children with behavioural symptoms in each age-group	6%	47%	42%	28%	34%

For both the first two questions, which were asked of all children, and also for the specific age group questions, the 3-5-year-olds appeared to present the most problems, especially difficulties in sleeping.   The 6-10-year-olds came next with school work problems and enuresis, followed by the 11-15-year-olds, whose main difficulties were again related to school work and also to friends.   The least troublesome seemed to be babies, who not only presented fewer difficulties of management but none of them showed marked delay in the early milestones of development.   These latter were perhaps the most diagnostic of the questions, whereas the remainder covered areas of perceived behavioural problems where normality is not clearly defined, let alone diagnosis.

The range of behaviour exhibited by children is very broad, and what might be considered unusual or alarming by some, may be viewed as perfectly normal by others.   In addition these questions were being asked of an adult about a child, and therefore like all children's symptoms whether physical or behavioural, were 'other-defined', unlike the symptoms of adults which were 'self-defined'. For instance, the following is an interviewer's comment on the 3-year-old son of a lamplighter: 'Parents said they take son's complaints with a pinch of salt, as he tends to imitate complaints he hears grown-ups make.'   The answers to questions about children therefore introduced the factor of the perception of the behaviour of one person by another, and depended on adult views of normality, which might vary widely and depend as much on personality as on cultural expectations.

Another factor in considering children's behaviour is the speed with which it can change as a child grows and adapts to new circumstances.   Most children can go through temporary 'bad' patches when quite 'normal' development may be seen as a nuisance or even as 'abnormal' by adults.   Figure 3.4 therefore shows the number of positive symptoms for the first two questions, expressed as a percentage of the number of children in each year.   These two questions

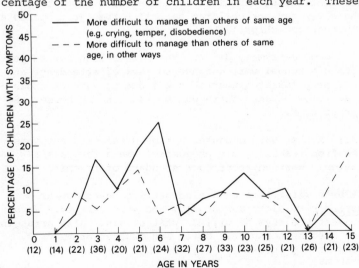

FIGURE 3.4   Management difficulties with children

on difficulties in management were asked about all children, and
positive responses to both rose at the ages of starting and leaving
school. One might expect things like crying, temper tantrums and
disobedience to be more common in young children, and these seemed
to reach their peak as primary school was started. Positive responses to both questions increased at, or just before, the change
from primary to secondary school. Finally, there was a marked rise
in other difficulties of management during adolescence and as
school leaving age was approached.

It is difficult to compare these findings with those of other
studies, because of the lack of any clear definitions for behavioural
symptoms in children. The methodology used here was practical and
pragmatic, but children's behavioural disorders present a very
diverse clinical picture.(69) Teachers and social workers may
perceive children's problems in very different ways,(70) and parents
may tend to normalize bizarre behaviour in their own offspring and
refrain from seeking help.(71) A recent study in Glasgow (72)
found that over half the children seen had one or more behavioural
problems which worried the mother, and similar proportions have been
reported from schools in America (73,74) with the prevalence among
boys being higher than girls as in the present study.

Undoubtedly, many behavioural problems in children were reflections of family backgrounds and difficulties at school, as the
following interviewers' comments illustrate:

14-year-old son of unemployed storeman: 'A problem family - father
won't work and younger brother is about to appear before the
Sheriff for rioting, assault and carrying offensive weapons.'

11-year-old son of labourer: 'Parents would have liked advice on how
to control other son aged nine. He had been in almost constant
trouble with the police for over a year - breaking and entering -
stealing and street fighting - malicious damage. She quite blithely
told me that she never fed her children herself - they just opened a
tin for themselves or got chips.'

9-year-old boy: 'House extremely dirty. The main reason for subject
being behind with his school work was due to lack of attendance at
school. Mother freely admitted that this was due to lack of shoes
or clothes, or at times because there was no food in the house. So
he was just kept at home.'

11-year-old girl: 'Mother said daughter a slow developer, but gets
no understanding from teacher, only prejudice. Need for parent-
teacher association. Worried about poor standard of teaching.'

34-year-old tailor's wife: 'Son aged nine getting beaten up at
school since moving here eight months ago, and very unhappy. Have
spoken to headmaster who says he will do what he can. Also arranging
for child to see speech therapist. Child had stutter previously.
Now so bad he can hardly speak.'

SOCIAL SYMPTOMS

Social symptoms were asked of adults only, and details of the
results are given in Appendix II. The four open-ended questions
were derived from the reasons for people presenting for social case
work at a family centre.(75) Apart from being graded for worry or
inconvenience, the answers were post-coded rather than being
categorized beforehand as for other symptoms. Almost a quarter of
all adults had at least one social symptom and 21 subjects gave
positive responses to all four questions.

The prevalence of the four main groups of social symptoms which
were causing worry or inconvenience, is also indicated in Appendix
II. In general, fewer symptoms in each group were graded as
causing moderate worry or inconvenience as were said to cause
slight or a lot of worry or inconvenience. Difficulties with other
members of the family or relatives produced the highest proportion
of a lot of worry or inconvenience, and boys seemed to cause more
worry than girls. The 6-10 and 16-20 year age-groups gave rise to
the most difficulties, and behavioural problems such as those associated with insomnia, disobedience and sex were the most frequent
reasons. Although specific illnesses and mental handicap appeared
as reasons for difficulties, there was no mention of physical handicap. It is perhaps surprising that problems with children and
teenagers should be the smallest group of social symptoms in view
of the origins of the Social Work 'Scotland' Act in the Kilbrandon
Report on children and young persons.(76) Husbands, wives and
grown-up children, followed by parents, were the other relatives
to cause most difficulties, especially young adult men and elderly
women. Marital relationships, often involving husbands' drinking,
caused considerable problems, as did illness and dependent relatives
especially elderly women.

Financial difficulties were the largest group of social symptoms,
although the definitions were subjective because in a sense almost
anyone could claim financial difficulties at some time - even the
wealthy on the grounds that they have more to lose. The post-coded
categories for income and expenditure difficulties were not
mutually exclusive, nor was the distinction between them always
clear. Nevertheless, unemployment (much of it long-term) emerged
as the major cause of low income, and the payment of rents and rates
as the main difficulty in expense. These were followed by the
problems of being on strike or illness, and the payment of specific
bills. It is interesting that official statistics showed that the
rate of financial assistance given by social work departments in
Glasgow was over twice that for Scotland as a whole.(77)

The last main group of social symptoms, for other difficulties or
problems with day-to-day life, was very broad indeed, as was the
explicit remit of the social work departments in Scotland.(78)
Housing caused by far the most problems and was at the root of other
social symptoms such as financial difficulties and worries about
elderly relatives. Disability or illness, and problems relating to
work were mentioned most frequently after housing in this group.
Although none of these other difficulties or problems with day-to-
day life had a duration of more than ten years, the majority were
long term and a matter of months and years, rather than a few weeks.

Overall then, the commonest specific social symptoms were financial difficulties and housing, followed by personal relationships
between adults, and behavioural disorders amongst children or teenagers. Alcoholism was probably understated, but emerged from
interviewers' comments such as 'Family rows due to heavy drinking'
(59-year-old housewife). Unemployment was also behind many social
problems, as illustrated by the following:

45-year-old labourer: 'On strike and very anxious about the lack of
money to keep home going. Has been unable to get any work. Is now
so depressed that he just lies in his bed most of the time.'

50-year-old unemployed production clerk: 'Very thoughtful man.
Former furnaceman prior to becoming clerk with diabetes. No bitter-
ness, but worry about employment.'

39-year-old unemployed storeman: 'Subject lost a good job and says
he can't get a comparable one in Glasgow area. Appears to have lost
heart. Goes fishing every day.'

Sometimes comments in the questionnaires indicated transient difficulties, for instance the 36-year-old wife of a scrap-dealer:
'"Bruises from fighting my man the other night" - but no residual
animosity.' But often there were situations where multiple problems
seemed to swamp individuals in insoluble situations, as the following
two extracts illustrate:

19-year-old wife of unemployed labourer: 'Living in conditions of
utmost squalor and overcrowding. Mother of respondent was being
savaged by her own dog during the interview. Respondent's sister
aged about seven, played in rubbish yard at the back, screaming
because she didn't want to go to school. Interview punctured by
shouted threats to her, and baby nursed by respondent was being
sick. Several people wandered in and out unannounced during interview. Altogether found by interviewer to be a stressful situation.
Front "garden" a mass of mud, rubbish and barbed wire. Respondent
pregnant and recently married. She was worried at prospect of
having baby at present abode, but no money, husband out of work,
and not even on Corporation waiting list.'

45-year-old staff nurse: 'A very nice woman who, as she says, seems
to be banging her head against a brick wall with every department
with which she is in touch. Is told that she will be all right
when divorce comes through, but no agency faces the problem of how
she exists in the meantime. Works three nights a week. Having
struggle with housing department, social security, factor and tax
authority. Has had nervous breakdown but went as out-patient to
hospital, rather than in-patient, because she couldn't leave her
children. Her main worries are - Divorce pending from alcoholic
husband, whom she is afraid of visiting her and has molested her
children. Fourteen year old son getting into wrong company. Lonely,
as mother just emigrated. Battling with taxation authorities.
Worried about tenancy of house and dangerous condition of electric
wiring, which the factor will not repair.'

It is difficult to compare the results for social symptoms found in
this survey with those of other studies because of differences in
methods and definitions. In a survey in Buckinghamshire (79) difficulties of adjustment to illness or disability, followed by personality problems, were found to be more common than inadequate means
or housing problems. In the same study a third of the social problems dealt with by general practitioners related to mental illness
or subnormality. A survey of general practice in Liverpool,(80)
however, reported that extreme poverty and housing were amongst the
commonest reasons for referral to an attached social worker. Such
results depend on the attitudes of doctors, who may know little of
social work and only refer for instance as a last resort in mental
illness.(81) In addition, the prevalence of social symptoms depends
on whether they are reported from the community or referred from
doctors. Family problems relating to marital difficulties or
children were twice as common as problems of finance or housing,
amongst cases referred to an attached social worker at a health
centre, and only 12 per cent had been previously known to a social
work department.(82) These findings emphasize the importance of
integrating social work and health care.(83)

SYMPTOM GRADINGS

Physical, mental and behavioural symptoms were considered together
as medical symptoms and were all graded for pain, disability, seriousness, and duration, as indicated in Appendix I. Social symptoms were
graded separately for worry or inconvenience. These gradings were
the subjective responses of those being interviewed and did not
involve value-judgments by another person. The scales were used in
two ways; first, to calculate mean scores for each subject, by
dividing the sum of each grading scale by the number of symptoms,
so that the mean score allowed for the differing numbers of symptoms
per person. The second use of the grading scales was to calculate
the mean referral and incongruous referral scores as defined in
Figure 1.4 and described in the next chapter. A subject with two
symptoms - one graded severe for pain (grade 3) and referred to a
doctor (grade 3 for professional referral), and the other causing
no pain (grade 1) but resulting in a request for advice from a
friend (grade 2 for lay referral) - would have a mean pain score of
$\frac{1}{2}(3 \times 1 + 1 \times 1) = 2$, and a mean referral score of $\frac{1}{2}(3 \times 1 + 2 \times 1) = 2.5$.
    Over one-third of subjects had at least one medical symptom for
which the pain or its equivalent was severe; 33 people said that all
their medical symptoms caused severe pain and one person had 18
symptoms so graded. About one-quarter of those interviewed had at
least one medical symptom for which the disability or inconvenience
was severe; 27 people said that all their medical symptoms caused
severe disability and one person graded 13 of his symptoms as
severe for disability. The majority of symptoms were not considered
to be serious, but 14 people thought that all their medical symptoms
were serious and 2 subjects had 9 symptoms so graded. There were
more subjects for whom the seriousness of symptoms was unknown than
in the previous two scales because this category was sometimes used
to indicate doubts about seriousness rather than lack of information,

whereas such doubts were intended to be graded as 'might be serious'.
The scale for worry or inconvenience referred to social symptoms and
was for adults only. Most adults reported no social symptoms or
considered that they caused no worry or inconvenience, but there
were 83 people with at least one social symptom which caused a lot
of worry or inconvenience.

TABLE 3.2 Duration of medical symptoms

Grading for the duration of medical symptoms		Number of subjects with one or more medical symptoms so graded
1 Symptom started) during past two) weeks and never) had before)	2 days or less	83 (6%)
	3 - 6 days	91 (7%)
	7 - 14 days	197 (15%)
2 Symptom started) during past two) weeks but had) before)	1 or 2 times	186 (14%)
	3 - 6 times	247 (18%)
	7 or more times	565 (42%)
3 Symptom started	2 - 12 weeks ago	386 (29%)
4 Symptom started	3 - 12 months ago	407 (30%)
5 Symptom started	1 - 5 years ago	584 (44%)
6 Symptom started	over 5 years ago	698 (52%)

Mean duration score	Number of subjects
0 - 0.9	162 (12%)
1.0 - 1.9	88 (7%)
2.0 - 2.9	228 (17%)
3.0 - 3.9	316 (24%)
4.0 - 4.9	326 (24%)
5.0 - 5.9	152 (11%)
6.0	72 (5%)
Total	1344 (100%)

The duration scale was designed to distinguish new symptoms from
those which were episodic, as well as indicating the duration of
symptoms. As shown in Table 3.2 more people had had fresh episodes
of previous symptoms than completely new symptoms in the previous
fortnight. Most subjects had chronic symptoms for some time, over
half of them having had at least one symptom for more than five
years. In all 72 people had had all their medical symptoms for
longer than five years and one person had 21 symptoms for this
length of time.

TABLE 3.3   Mean scores for symptom grading scales (1,344 subjects
for medical symptoms, and 964 adults for social symptoms)

Mean scores	Percentage of subjects for medical symptoms			Percentage of adults for social symptoms
	Pain	Disability	Seriousness	Worry
0 - 0.9	12	13	16	77
1.0 - 1.9	28	44	79	10
2.0 - 2.9	39	32	4	6
3.0 - 3.9	19	9	1	7
4.0	2	2	-	-

Table 3.3 shows the mean scores for each grading scale, except
for duration, expressed as grouped percentages. The scales for
perceived seriousness and worry did not go beyond three, but in
general the mean scores for pain tended to be higher than those for
disability or perceived seriousness. The grading scale for duration
in fact measured both periodicity and length of time, which made the
mean scores difficult to compare or interpret. Most symptoms seemed
to be either episodic or chronic. A longitudinal study in New York
(84) concluded that the mean duration of an illness in the community
was one week, but it would have required a follow-up to calculate a
mean duration from the present survey which only recorded a two-
week period prevalence. The mean grading scores did not increase
with the number of symptoms, and only the mean duration score gave
significant correlations with all the symptom frequencies. These
relationships were not, however, linear as there tended to be fewer
symptoms when the mean duration was within the previous two weeks or
for more than five years.

NUMBER OF SYMPTOMS PER PERSON

The information on individual symptoms was combined to give single
scores for the number of symptoms per person for each subject. There
were four such scores for each of the four main groups of symptoms -
physical symptoms for all ages, mental symptoms for adults, behavioural symptoms for children and social symptoms for adults. These
scores were used as the dependent variables for symptom prevalence,
if necessary regrouping data into categories of reasonable size for
correlations and multivariate analysis.

Of those interviewed 86 per cent had at least one physical symptom,
with a mean of 4.3 per person and a maximum of 25. The 14 per cent
with no physical symptoms was the same proportion as those who
reported no illnesses, injuries or disabilities in a community study
in Australia.(18) The Peckham Health Centre before the war found
that 12 per cent of their sample had no complaints,(7) as did a more
recent pilot study in London,(4) although this proportion was considerably reduced in the main survey which included mental symptoms. A

mean of about 4 physical symptoms per person was also found in
another recent study,(5) although the value of such comparisons is
limited by the very different research methods used.

Of adults 51 per cent had one or more mental symptoms, with a
mean of 1.1 per adult and a maximum of seven. Of the children 24
per cent and 23 per cent of the adults in the survey had behavioural
and social symptoms respectively, with a mean of 0.3 and a maximum
of 4 for both frequencies. The extent to which these findings compare with those of other studies has already been discussed, and
depends on the definitions and research methods used.

REFERENCES

1 Jones, F.A. (1972), 'Richard Asher Talking Sense', Pitman
   Medical, London.
2 Kirscht, J.P. (1971), Social and Psychological Problems of
   Surveys on Health and Illness, 'Social Science and Medicine,
   5, 519-26.
3 Crogono, A.W. (1973), Measurement of Ill-Health: A Comment,
   'International Journal of Epidemiology', 2, 5-6.
4 Wadsworth, M.E.J., Butterfield, W.J.H. and Blaney, R. (1971),
   'Health and Sickness: The Choice of Treatment', Tavistock,
   London.
5 Dunnell, K. and Cartwright, A. (1972), 'Medicine Takers,
   Prescribers and Hoarders', Routledge & Kegan Paul, London.
6 Rafibekov, S.D. (1969), Some Features of Morbidity, 'Sovet
   Zdravookhr', 28/12, 20-1.
7 Pearse, I.H. and Crocker, L.H. (1943), 'The Peckham Experiment',
   Allen & Unwin, London.
8 Morrell, D.C. (1970), Presenting Symptoms in General Practice,
   'British Journal of Preventive and Social Medicine', 24, 64.
9 Morrell, D.C. (1972), Symptom Interpretation in General Practice, 'Journal of the Royal College of General Practitioners',
   28/118, 297-309.
10 Murray Boyle, C. (1970), Differences between Doctors' and
   Patients' Interpretations of Common Medical Terms, 'British
   Medical Journal', 2/5704, 286-9.
11 Wittenborn, J.R. (1972), Reliability, Validity and Objectivity
   of Symptom-Rating Scales, 'Journal of Nervous and Mental
   Disease', 154/2, 79-87.
12 Cochrane, A.L. (1972), History of Measurement of Ill Health,
   'International Journal of Epidemiology', 1/2, 89-92.
13 Mayne, J.G. et al. (1969), A Health Questionnaire based on
   Paper-and-Pencil Medium, 'Journal of the American Medical
   Association', 208/11, 2064-8.
14 Elinson, J. and Trussell, R.E. (1957), Some Factors Relating to
   Degree of Correspondence for Diagnostic Information as Obtained
   by Household Interviews and Clinical Examination, 'American
   Journal of Public Health', 47, 311.
15 Meltzer, J.W. et al. (1970), Reliability and Validity of Survey
   Data on Physical Health, 'Public Health Reports', 85, 1075-86.
16 Kosa, J. et al. (1967), On the Reliability of Family Health
   Information, 'Social Science and Medicine', 1, 165-81.

17 Marquis, K.H. (1970), Effects of Social Reinforcement on Health
    Reporting in the Household Interview, 'Sociometry', 33, 203-15.
18 Bridges-Webb, C. (1974), The Traralgon Health and Illness
    Survey: Prevalence of Illness and Use of Health Care, 'Inter-
    national Journal of Epidemiology', 3, 37-46.
19 Koos, E.L. (1954), 'The Health of Regionville', Columbia Univer-
    sity Press, New York.
20 Office of Health Economics (1972), 'Medicine and Society',
    London.
21 Kennedy, T.M. (1973), Annual report from Langholm general
    practice 1971, 'Update' 6/9, 1285-1300.
22 Scottish Standing Medical Advisory Committee (1973), 'The
    Future of Chest Services in Scotland', HMSO, Edinburgh.
23 Rose, G.A. (1962), The Diagnosis of Ischaemic Heart Pain and
    Intermittent Claudication in Field Surveys, 'Bulletin of the
    World Health Organisation', 27, 645-58.
24 Milne, J.S. and Williamson, J. (1972), The Use of Medical
    Services by Older People, 'Health Bulletin', 31/4, 263-8.
25 Christian, W. (1969), Frequency of Disease and Accidents in
    German Federal Republic in April, 1966, 'Off. Gesundh. Wes',
    31/1, 23-38.
26 Bakken, A.F. (1971), Experiences of the General Practitioner
    in Oslo, January - April 1970, 'T. Norske Laegeforen', 91/3,
    215-18.
27 Langholm Health Centre (1968), 'Annual Report'.
28 Office of Health Economics (1973), 'Rheumatism and Arthritis in
    Britain', London.
29 Office of Health Economics (1973), 'Skin Disorders', London.
30 Wood, M.M. and Elwood, P.C. (1966), Symptoms of Iron Deficiency
    Anaemia, 'British Journal of Preventive and Social Medicine',
    20, 117-21.
31 Kilpatrick, G.S. (1969), 'The Early Diagnosis of Anaemia',
    Office of Health Economics, London.
32 Robinson, J.O. and Wood, M.M. (1968), Symptoms and Personality
    in the Diagnosis of Physical Illness, 'British Journal of Pre-
    ventive and Social Medicine', 22, 23-6.
33 Barolin, G.S. and Schnaberth, G. (1972), Two Year Report of an
    Austrian Headache Centre, 'Wein. Klein Wschr.', 84/8, 126-30.
34 Foulds, G.A. and Hope, K. (1968), 'Manual of the Symptom-Sign
    Inventory', University of London Press.
35 Derogatis, L.R. (1974), The Hopkins Symptom Checklist (HSCL),
    A Self-Report Symptom Inventory, 'Behavioural Science', 19, 1.
36 Goldberg, D.P. et al. (1970), Standardised Psychiatric Interview
    for Use in Community Studies, 'British Journal of Preventive and
    Social Medicine', 24, 18-23.
37 Kupfer, D.J. et al. (1972), Scale for Symptom Discrimination,
    'Psychology Reports', 30, 915.
38 Semmence, A.M. (1969), The Health Opinion Survey. A Psychiatric
    Screening Instrument, 'Journal of the Royal College of General
    Practitioners', 18, 344-8.
39 Summers, G.F. (1971), Cross Validation of Questions with a
    Rural Sample, 'Rural Sociology', 36, 367.
40 'British Medical Journal' (1970), The Language of Illness, 1,
    768-9.

41 Berndt, H. (1968), The Sociogenesis of Mental Symptoms, 'Soziale
    Welt', 191, 22-46.
42 Timms, N. (1967), 'A Sociological Approach to Social Problems',
    Routledge & Kegan Paul, London.
43 Grunt, M. (1973), Aspects of Informal Labelling and Sanctions for
    Mentally Deviant Behaviour, 'Kolner Zeitschrift fur Soziologie
    und Sozial-Psychologie', 25/2, 365-85.
44 Goffman, E. (1969), The Insanity of Place, 'Psychiatry', 32/4,
    357-88.
45 Weinstein, R.M. (1972), Patients' Perceptions of Mental Illness,
    'Journal of Health and Social Behaviour', 13, 38-47.
46 Downey, K.J. (1967), Public Image of Mental Illness, 'Social
    Science and Medicine', 1, 45-65.
47 Piedmont, E.B. and Downey, K.J. (1971), Revolutions in Psychiatry,
    'International Journal of Social Psychology', 17/2, 111-21.
48 Reinhardt-Schnadt, H. (1973), People's Attitudes Towards the
    Mentally Ill, 'Kolner Zeitschrift fur Soziologie und Sozial-
    Psychologie', 25/2, 336-49.
49 Jordan, J.M. et al. (1973), Community Attitudes to Mental
    Illness, 'Medical Journal of Australia', 1, 729-33.
50 Kleiner, R.J. and Seymour, P. (1971), Potential Sources of Error
    in Epidemiological Surveys of Mental Illness, 'International
    Journal of Social Psychiatry', 17/2, 122-32.
51 Klein, D.C. (1968), 'Community Dynamics and Mental Health',
    John Wiley, New York.
52 Agras, S. et al. (1969), Epidemiology of Common Fears and
    Phobias, 'Comprehensive Psychiatry', 10/2, 151-6.
53 Central Statistical Office (1973), 'Social Trends No.4', HMSO,
    London.
54 Goldberg, D.P. and Blackwell, B. (1970), Psychiatric Illness in
    General Practice, 'British Medical Journal', 5707, 439-43.
55 Bebbington, R. (1969), Review of 508 Consecutive Patients seen
    in General Practice, 'Journal of the Royal College of General
    Practitioners', 18/84, 27-37.
56 Lonnguist, J. and Niskanen, P. (1973), Psychiatric Disturbance
    in Helsinki, 'Psychiat. Fenn.', 279-83.
57 Giel, R. (1972), Psychiatry in General Practice, 'Huisarts
    Wetensch', 15/6, 203-9.
58 Parker, G. (1972), Psychiatric Morbidity, 'Medical Journal of
    Australia', 1/19, 993-6.
59 Cormack, J.J. (1971), One Year's Practice, 'Practitioner',
    207/1238, 230-5.
60 Cooper, B. (1972), Clinical and Social Aspects of Chronic
    Neurosis, 'Practitioner', 208, 289-90.
61 Rawnsley, K. (1968), 'The Early Diagnosis of Depression', Office
    of Health Economics, London.
62 Downing, R.W. (1974), Mixed Anxiety - Depression', 'Archives of
    General Psychiatry', 30, 312-17.
63 Kellner, R. (1972), Relationship of Depressive Neurosis to
    Anxiety and Somatic Symptoms, 'Psychosomatic', 13/6, 358-62.
64 Maxwell, A.E. (1973), Psychiatric Illnesses and Symptomatology,
    'British Journal of Psychiatry', 122, 251.
65 Carpenter, W.J. and Strauss, J.S. (1974), First Rank Symptoms in
    Schizophrenia, 'American Journal of Psychiatry', 131/6, 682-7.

66 Kay, D.W. et al. (1969), Factor Analysis of Mental Symptoms,
    'British Journal of Psychiatry', 115, 377-88.
67 Demel, I. (1973), Multivariate Analysis of Psychic and Somatic
    Symptoms in Depression, 'Psychotherapeutics Psychosomatics',
    22, 121-30.
68 Stone, F.H. (1971), Personal communication.
69 Wollf, S. (1971), Symptoms in Disturbed Children, 'British
    Journal of Psychiatry', 118/545, 421-7.
70 Jones, D.G. (1969), Attitudes of Social Workers and Teachers
    to Children's Behaviour Problems, 'Social Work', 26/4, 12-13.
71 Pritchard, C. (1972), An Analysis of Parental Attitudes towards
    the Treatment of Maladjusted Children, 'British Journal of
    Social Work', 2, 69-81.
72 Ford, L.R. (1973), 'The Community's Unmet Child Health Needs',
    Dissertation, University of Glasgow.
73 Werry, J.S. and Quay, H.C. (1971), Behavioural Symptoms and
    Young Children, 'Am. J. Orth.', 41, 136.
74 Mumford, E. (1972), Physical, Social and Emotional Problems in
    an Elementary School, 'Paper at 3rd International Conference of
    Social Science and Medicine - Elsinore'.
75 Maddox, E.J. (1971), Analysis of some data from the Drumchapel
    Family Centre, Unpublished paper.
76 Scottish Home and Health Department (1964), 'Children and Young
    Persons in Scotland', HMSO, Edinburgh.
77 Social Work Services Group (1974), 'Scottish Social Work
    Statistics 1972', Scottish Education Department, HMSO, Edinburgh.
78 Scottish Education Department and Scottish Home & Health
    Department (1966), 'Social Work and the Community', HMSO,
    Edinburgh.
79 Jefferys, M. (1965), 'An Anatomy of Social Welfare Services',
    Michael Joseph, London.
80 Ratoff, L. and Pearson, B. (1970), Social Casework in General
    Practice: An Alternative Approach, 'British Medical Journal',
    2/570, 475-7.
81 Roy, R.G. (1967), A Short Study of Community Care Cases Referred
    by General Practitioners, 'Social Work', 24/3, 3-8.
82 Willis, M. (1973), Social Work, 'Health Bulletin', 31/3, 144.
83 Cowin, R. (1970), Some New Dimensions of Social Work Practice
    in a Health Setting, 'American Journal of Public Health', 60/5,
    860-9.
84 Lebowitz, M.D. et al. (1972), Duration of Minor Illness,
    'American Review of Respiratory Disease', 106/6, 835-41.

Chapter 4

PATTERNS OF REFERRAL

'The happiness and unhappiness of the rational social animal depends
not on what he feels, but on what he does.'

Marcus Aurelius (AD 121-80)

The action taken by someone in response to his symptoms, or those of
a child, is referral behaviour which might be a positive action, or
negative, that is, absence of action. The referral behaviour for
medical and social symptoms is first described, followed by the
results of the computed referral scores. These scores were calculated by ranking the different types of referral and allowing for
the varying numbers of symptoms per person as indicated in Figure
1.3. In this way patterns of referral were identified which
indicated the tendency for someone to refer symptoms formally, and
the extent to which a person contributed to the symptom 'iceberg'
or 'trivia'.

REFERRAL OF MEDICAL SYMPTOMS

All positive symptoms were coded for source of referral. Medical
symptoms consisted of physical symptoms for all subjects, mental
symptoms for adults, and behavioural symptoms for children. The
referral of all these was pre-coded according to the same ranking
scale (see Appendix I), and the frequencies of referral for these
types of symptoms are shown in Appendix III. Each subject could
have several symptoms which might be referred in different ways,
but if a single symptom had been referred in more than one way,
then it was coded for the most formal referral. Of the referrals
coded as 'other', many were to a chemist for physical symptoms, and
some for behavioural symptoms were to teachers.
   The majority of subjects did nothing about most of their
physical symptoms, although almost half took at least some to their
doctors. But 15 per cent asked members of their family about such
symptoms, and 10 per cent took specific physical symptoms directly
to dentist, chiropodists or opticians. Very few physical symptoms
were referred to friends, or to nurses or health visitors, but

about 5 per cent of people took physical symptoms directly to a
hospital casualty or outpatient department. A much smaller proportion of subjects referred mental or behavioural symptoms to a
doctor.

It is difficult to make a direct comparison between the
frequencies of referral for these three types of medical symptoms,
because a different proportion of subjects had positive symptoms in
each category. Eighty-six per cent had at least one physical
symptom, 51 per cent of adults had one or more mental symptoms, and
24 per cent of children had behavioural symptoms. Table 4.1 takes
account of these different proportions by expressing the referrals
as the percentage of those who had positive symptoms. It can be
seen that people were much more likely to take physical symptoms to
a doctor than mental or behavioural symptoms. The majority of
medical symptoms were not referred at all, but inaction was least
likely for children's behavioural symptoms.

TABLE 4.1   Comparison of medical referrals

Type of referral	% of subjects with positive symptoms		
	All subjects' physical	Adult mental	Children's behavioural
Not known	1	1	1
Nobody	84	85	58
Family or relative	18	14	14
Friend or acquaintance	1	2	0
Nurse or health visitor	1	0	0
Dentist, chiropodist, optician	11	0	0
Own GP, partner or locum	51	25	21
Hospital doctor in casualty or OP	5	< 1	0
Other	6	< 1	19
Total number of subjects with positive symptoms	1157	492	90

Recent estimates of the extent of self-treatment in the United
Kingdom have varied from three-quarters of all symptoms,[1] to half
the patients in general practice.[2] Many of these may have been
minor illnesses, which according to one review [3] comprise almost
two-thirds of the work of family doctors, although the cumulative
impact of minor illnesses in terms of sickness absence may be considerable.[4] A study in London [5] reported that 26 per cent of
those interviewed had formally referred their complaints for medical advice, which is much less than the proportion found for

physical symptoms in the present survey.   But the London study included mental symptoms amongst complaints, whereas these were considered separately here.   This may have been partly why mental symptoms were not found to be markedly less likely to be referred to a doctor in London, where complaints such as tiredness were classified as mental symptoms.

REFERRAL OF SOCIAL SYMPTOMS

The referral of social symptoms is considered separately from the three types of medical symptoms, because social symptom referral was post-coded by tabulating the answers from two months of the survey and constructing categories on the basis of this information. The referral of social symptoms seemed to be of two distinct sorts, one informal and the other formal involving specific professions or agencies.   The results for these two types of referral were coded independently and are shown in Appendix III.

Approximately half the referrals for social symptoms were informal, of which the great majority consisted of doing nothing, and the other half were formal referrals.   When people said that they had done nothing about a symptom, an attempt was made to find out why.   Some said they felt powerless or helpless to do anything, and others gave a more specific reason for doing nothing, such as depression.   Most of those who took some positive action about a situation did so on their own, and for a few this implied avoiding certain circumstances or people.

The most frequent formal action was to go to the Social Security Office or Employment Exchange, which included referrals for unemployment benefit.   This was followed by referrals to a doctor or hospital, and to the category of 'other', which included the police, lawyers, tenants' associations, and councillors.   During the whole survey only one person was mentioned by name as a source of formal social referral, and that was a local councillor who held regular advice sessions.   Few people referred themselves to a social worker or social work department for social symptoms, and only one each to a minister or nurse.   About twice as many subjects referred social symptoms to factors or the housing department, as did to social workers, who only accounted for about 4 per cent of all such formal referrals.   It may have been that the social security or housing departments were appropriate sources of advice, but these findings indicate that the medical profession was much more likely to be seen as a source of referral for social problems than the social work profession whose role seemed rather peripheral.

TENDENCY TO REFER FORMALLY

As individuals had different numbers of symptoms which were referred in a variety of ways, it was necessary to take these factors into account in order to calculate a single score for each person which indicated their tendency to seek formal advice about symptoms.   It was also necessary to have two such composite referral scores, because all the medical symptoms (physical, mental and behavioural)

had been pre-coded separately from the social symptoms, which were
post-coded. Both medical and social symptom referrals were first
grouped into three broad categories as shown in Table 4.2, which
provided a conceptual ranking scale. Mean referral scores were
then calculated for each subject as defined in Figure 1.4. There
were two such scores, one for medical symptoms and the other for
social symptoms, which were simply the sum of a person's referral
rank orders divided by the number of symptoms he had.

TABLE 4.2 Grouping of medical and social referrals

Score	Category	Medical referral	Social referral
1	None	Nobody	Nothing because felt powerless or helpless Nothing because of other specific reason Avoidance Self
2	Lay or informal	Family or relative Friend or acquaintance	Informal through relative Informal through friend Informal through other source or combination of informal
3	Professional or formal	Nurse or health visitor Dentist, chiropodist, optician (direct) Own GP, partner or locum Hospital doctors in casualty or outpatients (direct)	Doctor/hospital Nurse/health visitor Social worker/social work dept./ medical social worker Teacher Minister/priest Factor/housing dept. Social security/ employment exchange Other formal source

The frequency distributions of these mean referral scores are
given in Table 4.3. Subjects who had no symptoms could not have a
mean referral score, nor could those who had symptoms for which no
referral was known. This latter factor accounts for the fact that
fewer subjects had mean referral scores than had symptoms, particularly for social symptoms. The results suggest a lack of formal
referral for medical symptoms, and the opposite tendency for social
symptoms.
    Conceptually, the three broad referral categories of none, lay
and professional for medical symptoms, are equivalent to the categories of none, informal and formal for social symptoms. It is
therefore feasible to compare the referral of the three types of
medical symptoms and the social symptoms. This is done in Figure 4.1

TABLE 4.3   Frequency of mean referral scores

Mean medical referral score

$$= \frac{\text{Sum of physical, mental and behavioural symptom referral scores}}{\text{Number of physical, mental and behavioural symptoms}}$$

Mean medical referral score	Number of subjects
1.0 to < 1.5	513
1.5 to < 2.0	246
2.0 to < 2.5	246
2.5 to < 3.0	60
3.0	78

Mean social referral score

$$= \frac{\text{Sum of social symptom referral scores}}{\text{Number of social symptoms}}$$

Mean social referral score	Number of adults
1.0 to < 2.0	53
2.0 to < 3.0	23
3.0	82

by expressing the results in terms of proportions of symptoms rather than subjects, any one of whom might refer a number of symptoms in different ways.

It seems that people were least likely to do anything about mental symptoms followed by children's behavioural symptoms. In a recent study in America (6) it was found that the great majority of subjects had had contact with someone who was mentally ill, of whom over two-thirds had sought help themselves. Although mental symptoms are not the same as mental illness, it may be that psychiatric disorders are more recognized and accepted in America than Scotland.

About one-fifth of the behavioural symptoms in children were referred informally; apart from this there was little evidence of any extensive lay referral system for other types of symptoms. One might expect advice to be sought for children's behavioural problems from friends and relatives. In a recent survey in Glasgow (7) only 2 per cent of behaviour worries in children were seen by mothers as reasons for going to the family doctor. Lay referral may be more significant where there is more 'shopping around' for medical care, and a study of the elderly in America,(8) showed the importance of informal networks for information about doctors.

These scores did not record the reasons for particular actions

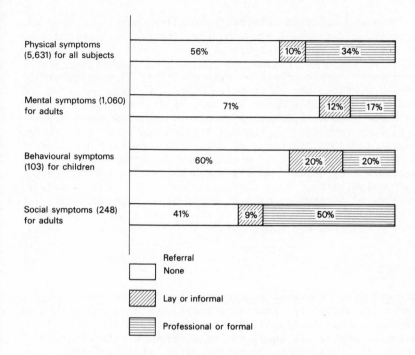

FIGURE 4.1   Referral for main groups of symptoms

being taken, which obviously depended on individual situations.   For
instance, some parents might be more likely to take children to
doctors than themselves, as illustrated by the following:

8-year-old daughter of office clerk: 'Mother would go to doctor
about something wrong with children, as you can't tell if it is
serious or not; wouldn't go for herself until she had seen how it
developed.'

Sometimes reluctance to refer symptoms for professional advice
seemed to stem from either fear or ignorance, which were rationalized
in passing comments such as the following:

4-year-old son of a plasterer: 'Mother had had a lump for six
months; will go soon to the doctor, but would be taking someone
else's place when there.   Seemed very reluctant to trouble the
doctor.'

55-year-old wife of a cabinet maker: 'Coughed up blood - just a wee
bit.   Didn't think to mention it when down at doctor's a few days
later.'

No action was taken for over half the physical symptoms, of which
about one-third were referred for professional advice, mainly to
doctors.   It is interesting that social symptoms were much the most
likely to be formally referred, although very few of them to social
workers.   These findings are in contrast to those of a survey in San

Francisco,(9) where delay in referral, and self-coping, appeared to
be more pronounced for social symptoms than for mental symptoms, and
were least likely for physical symptoms.

Apart from differences in time and place, such comparisons are
tenuous because of varying research methods. This is particularly
true of social symptoms for which definitions are hazy, and what one
person thinks is a social symptom may be very different from the
views of another. Quite apart from research, social workers may
perceive problems in terms of personal adjustments over time, while
clients may be looking for practical help with immediate difficulties.(10) Although the remit of social work departments is very
broad, there are many other formal sources for such practical help,
as this survey indicates. The difficulties of definition, however,
do not invalidate research or make it meaningless. Rather they
reflect the lack of clarity in service objectives and re-emphasize
the need for a critical and constructive evaluation of social work.

'ICEBERGS' AND 'TRIVIA'

The symptom gradings described in the previous chapter were combined
with the referral scores in order to identify subjects who were not
taking symptoms for professional advice when perhaps they should
have done so, or conversely those who were formally referring
symptoms when this appeared to be unnecessary. This begs the
question of when symptoms need or do not need professional attention.
It was here that the symptom gradings were used, because like the
positive responses to questions about symptoms, the answers were
entirely subjective and no attempt was made by the interviewers to
assess symptoms objectively or to grade them.

It seemed reasonable for someone not to seek professional advice
for symptoms which they themselves did not score at all on any of
the symptom gradings. Equally it was understandable for someone to
refer formally symptoms which they themselves scored highly on one
or more of these gradings. The implication is that the way in which
people experience symptoms has at least some bearing on what they do
about them. However, if a subject's own perception of a symptom
appeared to have little relevance to his referral behaviour, and
indeed was contrary to what might have been expected, then factors
other than the symptom itself would seem to have been determining
what action was taken. The term incongruous referral was therefore
used. This did not imply a value-judgment about what people should
do, but rather that what they actually did about a symptom did not
follow from how they themselves said they experienced the symptom.

It seemed important to identify such people, because for medical
symptoms some light might be thrown on the 'illness iceberg' (11) in
the community on the one hand, and on those who go to doctors with
'trivia' on the other hand. The analogy could be extended to social
symptoms, in order to see the extent to which formal agencies (of
which social work departments are only one) 'fit' the perceived
problems of people in the community. Because social symptoms were
graded differently from medical symptoms (physical, mental and
behavioural), it was necessary to have separate incongruous referral
scores for medical and social symptoms. These operationalized the

concepts of 'icebergs' and 'trivia' in a way which did not involve value-judgments about whether professional referral was appropriate or not. The only objective decisions concerned the cut-off points used for the symptom gradings. In the event these were as rigorous as possible, so that only those whose referral behaviour seemed inexplicable in terms of their own assessments of their symptoms, had incongruous referral scores.

These incongruous referral scores are defined in Figure 1.4. Twenty-three per cent of all subjects had at least one physical, mental or behavioural symptom for which they did not seek professional advice, although they said that the pain or disability was severe, or they thought the symptom was serious. One person had fifteen such symptoms. The social symptom 'iceberg' appeared to be much smaller, with 4 per cent of adults having one or two social symptoms for which they did not seek formal help, although they said that a lot of worry or inconvenience was being caused.

There have been several surveys looking at hidden morbidity in the community, not only in the United Kingdom,(5,12) but also in other countries.(13,14) A cross-cultural study of medical care utilization in America, Britain, and Yugoslavia (15) reported much the same patterns of primary care utilization irrespective of differences in the number of doctors, or in reported morbidity and disability. There were, however, considerable differences in hospital referral patterns. But these studies did not really define which symptoms or 'illnesses' were appropriate for medical referral, and certainly not by reference to the subjective perceptions of the subjects themselves.

Almost 10 per cent of those interviewed had at least one medical symptom for which they sought professional advice, although they said that there was no pain or disability, and that they did not think the symptom was serious. The maximum score for one subject was five medical symptoms referred for medical advice when there appeared to be no good reason for doing so. The equivalent social symptom 'trivia' were fewer than this, with only 3 per cent of adults referring one or two social symptoms for professional advice when they said that only slight worry or inconvenience was being caused.

A theme of recent conferences on health care has been the desire of professional groups to be rid of what they describe as 'trivia' to others.(16) One study of general practice in Britain (17) concluded that frustration lowered the quality of care, and was related to work load and professional attitudes, rather than to practice organization or factors such as background and education of doctors. There have been many surveys of work load in primary medical care from a number of countries,(18,19,20,21,22) but none of these seemed to take into account the quality of the demand. One study of health referral patterns in America (23) reported that 8 per cent of medical referrals were 'inappropriate' and a follow-up of patients in Germany (24) concluded that 11 per cent of the conditions seen were 'trifling'. But the criteria used in reaching these decisions did not appear to assess the perceptions of patients.

Although described together, the incongruous medical and social referral scores are not directly comparable because medical referrals were for all ages, whereas social referrals were for adults only.

Also, the criteria used to define an incongruous professional referral for social symptoms were less stringent than for medical symptoms
because the minimum grading for social symptoms was 'slight' whereas
that for medical symptoms was 'none'. In addition, the proportion
of adults with social symptoms was much smaller than the proportion
of all subjects with medical symptoms.

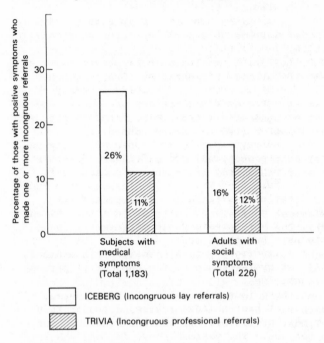

FIGURE 4.2   'Icebergs' and 'trivia'

In order to allow for this the numbers of subjects with incongruous referral scores are expressed in Figure 4.2 as a percentage
of those with positive symptoms. When compared in this way, the
amount of incongruous referral was not dissimilar for both medical
and social symptoms, with more people not seeking professional
advice when they probably should have done, than the other way
round. In particular, the extent of incongruous medical lay referrals suggests that the hidden 'illness iceberg' was about two-and-a-
half times the size of possible 'trivia' which found their way to
doctors. There did not appear to have been the same difference
between the 'iceberg' and 'trivia' for social symptoms. Similar
conclusions were reached by a study in Sweden,(25) which reported
that the ratio of met to unmet medical need was 1 : 1 whereas the
equivalent ratio for social need was 5 : 3.

This supports the impression of the present study that there was
more unmet medical than social need in the community as indicated
by figure 4.2. However, such statements need to be qualified by
consideration of the research methods used, which may vary considerably, especially for definitions of need and the nature of social
symptoms. In particular, referral behaviour is a complex process
which takes place over time, and the same person may behave quite

differently depending on the symptoms involved. For instance, in the present survey, incongruous lay and professional medical referrals were not mutually exclusive, and 7 per cent of those who were part of the 'iceberg' also referred 'trivia'.

REFERENCES

1   'Journal of the Royal College of General Practitioners' (1973), Self Care, Report 16, 7-9.
2   Elliott-Binns, C.P. (1973), An Analysis of Lay Medicine, 'Journal of the Royal College of General Practitioners', 23, 255-64.
3   'Journal of the Royal College of General Practitioners' (1973), Nature and Content of General Practice, Report 16, 24-8.
4   Office of Health Economics (1964), 'New Frontiers in Health', London.
5   Wadsworth, M.E.J., Butterworth, W.J.H. and Blaney, R. (1971), 'Health and Sickness: The Choice of Treatment', Tavistock, London.
6   Spiro, H.R. et al. (1974), The Issue of Contact with the Mentally Ill, 'American Journal of Public Health', 64, 876-9.
7   Ford, L.R. (1973), 'The Community's Unmet Child Health Needs', Dissertation, University of Glasgow.
8   Booth, A and Babchuck, N. (1972), Seeking Health Care from New Resources, 'Journal of Health and Social Behaviour', 13/1, 90-9.
9   Blackwell, B.L. (1967), Upper Middle Class Adult Expectation about Entering the Sick Role for Physical and Psychiatric Dysfunction, 'Journal of Health and Social Behaviour', 8, 83-95.
10 Mayer, J.E. and Timms, N. (1970), 'The Client Speaks', Routledge & Kegan Payl, London.
11 Last, J.M. (1963), The Illness Iceberg, 'Lancet', 6 July, 28-31.
12 Pearse, I.H. and Crocker, L.H. (1943), 'The Peckham Experiment', Allen & Unwin, London.
13 Van der Velden, H.G.M. (1973), Manifested and Hidden Morbidity in Housewives, 'T. Soc. Geneesk', 51/4, 140-4.
14 Iwanow, K.P. (1969), Requirements of the Population of an Urban Medical Region for Out-patient Health Care, 'Zdrow. Publ.', 80/10, 893-904.
15 White, K.L. and Murnagham, J.H. (1969), 'International Comparisons of Medical Care Utilization', US Department of Health, Education & Welfare, Washington DC.
16 Dopson, L. (1973), Trivia - the Threat to General Practice, 'Pulse', 27/6, 1.
17 Mechanic, D. (1970), Correlates of Frustration among British General Practitioners, 'Journal of Health and Social Behaviour', 11/2, 87-104.
18 Bogatziew, I.D. (1969), General Morbidity in an Urban Population and the Methods for Determining Normal Demands for Medical Care, 'Zdrow. Publ.', 80/10, 883-92.
19 McFarlane, A.H. and O'Connell, B.Q. (1969), Morbidity in Family Practice, 'Canadian Medical Association Journal', 101/5, 259-63.
20 Bernstein, J.M. and Dolan, L.J. (1972), Annual Reports from General Practice, 1970, 'Update', 4/8, 993-1004.

21   Meredith, H.C. (1972), Work Load and Morbidity in a Country
     General Practice, 'New Zealand Medical Journal', 76/485, 247-51.
22   Ridley Smith, R.M. (1973), Why the Patients Came, 'New Zealand
     Medical Journal', 79/499, 240-6.
23   Cauffman, J.G. et al. (1974), A Study of Health Referral
     Patterns, 'American Journal of Public Health', 64, 331-56.
24   Wesiack, W. (1971), Problems and Methods of Follow-up Examina-
     tions in Practice, 'Munch. Med. Wschr.', 113/28, 1023-8.
25   'Lancet' (1974), The Patients We Don't See, 7887, 995.

Chapter 5

USE AND PERCEPTION
OF MEDICAL SERVICES

'In particular no comprehensive or continuing information is available about who use general practitioner services and the way in which they are used.'   (Social Trends, 1970, HMSO)

The use of primary care is reflected in the amount of contact between the providers and recipients of services. This contact depends partly on the ease of access which may be indirect for instance by telephone, or direct by personal travel. The use of services will also be affected by how people perceive professionals such as doctors, and facilities like health centres. But there are other aspects of medical care which complement the work of general practitioners. One of these is the use of unprescribed as well as prescribed medicines. Another important aspect of primary care is the provision of family planning which may involve ordinary shops and special clinics, as well as family doctors.

CONTACT WITH PRIMARY CARE

Table 5.1 shows the number of surgery and home visits, made by subjects during the past year. Almost one-third had not seen their family doctor, partner, or locum in his surgery during the previous twelve months, but a small number had been more than twelve times during that period and could be called frequent attenders. One-quarter of those interviewed had had a home visit during the previous year, but few had been visited more than two or three times.
    It was not possible to calculate exact consultation rates because the questions on surgery and home visits were asked in a grouped form. However, by taking a mean value for the grouped categories, and assuming that the mean of the highest category was two visits more than its minimum, it was possible to make a reasonable estimate of the number of surgery and home visits per person per year. Using this method the results from the survey gave a rate for surgery visits of 2.6 per person per year, and for home visits of 0.6 per person per year. The two sets of figures combined gave a

TABLE 5.1   Surgery and home visits

Number of visits during past year	Number of subjects (%)	
	Surgery visits	Home visits
Not known	10 (1%)	14 (1%)
None	433 (32%)	1004 (75%)
1	287 (21%)	182 (14%)
2 or 3	313 (23%)	86 (6%)
4 to 6	159 (12%)	34 (2%)
7 to 12	89 (7%)	15 (1%)
13 or more	53 (4%)	9 (1%)
Total	1344 (100%)	1344 (100%)

consultation rate of 3.3 per person per year.

The rate for surgery visits was similar to those reported recently from the north of England (1) and from a new town in Scotland.(2)   Home visits comprised 18 per cent of the total consultation rate; this was less than the range given by a review of consultation rates in the United Kingdom over the past thirty years,(3) which showed considerable variations.   In general, consultation rates appear to have been declining in Britain,(4,5) with one survey (6) concluding that the trend of recent studies indicated a fall by 15 per cent in surgery visits and 60 per cent in home visits over the past twenty years.

The figures from the present survey were if anything on the low side, especially for home visits, when compared with other studies from the United Kingdom.   They were also lower than the annual consultation rates of about four per person found by studies from America,(7) Australia,(8) and the Netherlands.(9)   Such comparisons may be misleading because the consultation rates given may include direct visits to hospitals and telephone calls.   The study from America (7) indicated that 12 per cent of all medical consultations were by phone, which is about three times the figure given by the General Household Survey for the United Kingdom;(10) this same source also concluded that the annual consultation rates, including telephone conversations, were higher for Scotland than for England and Wales.

In some instances efforts to reduce the amount of house calls produced reactions from patients as illustrated by the following comments:

81-year-old widower: 'Would not call doctor out unless absolutely necessary. Has seen him only twice in eight years. Disgusted at recent leaflet about helping doctors.'

9-year-old son of sales representative: 'Parents complained of doctor's campaign against home visits, especially at night – makes you feel guilty about even calling.'

59-year-old corporation official: 'Doctors unwilling to come to
house. People won't call own doctor, but wait for night emergency
doctors. Patients bring babies direct to hospital rather than call
out doctor.'

TABLE 5.2 How doctor contacted

Method of contacting doctor	Number of respondents (%)
Not known or Don't know	14 (1%)
Attend health centre without appointment	19 (1%)
Attend health centre to make appointment	137 (10%)
Telephone doctor directly	32 (3%)
Telephone health centre for appointment	1070 (80%)
Get friend or relative to telephone	40 (3%)
Get friend or relative to call and make appointment	19 (1%)
Other	13 (1%)
Total	1344 (100%)

    Table 5.2 shows how those interviewed contacted their doctor.
Over 80 per cent used the telephone to make contact, the great
majority via an appointment at the health centre, with only a small
number telephoning their doctor directly. Some 10 per cent went to
the health centre themselves, and a few attended without an appointment. About 5 per cent got someone else to make the appointment,
and no one wrote letters. Clearly the telephone was the main means
of first making contact with primary medical care, but not for
telephone consultations as such, which appear to be much commoner
in America,(11) for instance for reporting symptoms.(12) As one
42-year-old housewife put it: 'No difficulty in contacting health
centre but no contact can be made directly with general practitioner
by phone. Not available outside health centre hours. Can't get
advice by phone.'
    Problems with the telephone were the main cause of difficulties
in contacting a doctor as indicated by Table 5.3, although most
people said that they had no difficulty in seeing or contacting
their doctor or the health centre. Those who did not have their
own telephone had to use someone else's or a public callbox, and
there were several complaints about public telephones being out of
order because of vandalism. The importance of the telephone and
also of receptionists was also emphasized by another study of
patients' views of a health centre in the United Kingdom.(13)
Those who had difficulty in contacting a doctor tended to have

TABLE 5.3   Difficulty in contacting doctor

Difficulty in contacting doctor	Number of respondents (%)
Not known	151 (11%)
None	960 (71%)
Difficulty in phoning health centre - public phone	89 (7%)
- someone else's phone	69 (5%)
Difficulty at reception/getting put through to doctor	30 (2%)
Difficulty in getting doctor/ waiting a long time	16 (1%)
Other reasons	20 (2%)
Combination of reasons	9 (1%)
Total	1344 (100%)

higher symptom frequencies and were more likely to seek professional advice. This suggests that referral behaviour proceded the difficulties in contacting a doctor rather than such difficulties determining referral behaviour.

To reach the health centre 55 per cent came by bus, but 27 per cent walked, with 12 per cent coming by car or taxi, and only 1 per cent by train. Over three-quarters of all those interviewed were within twenty minutes of the health centre, and 90 per cent were within forty minutes travelling time, with only two people taking more than an hour to get there. The health centre was therefore well placed for access, with most patients either living near a bus route or within walking distance. These two factors of method of travel and time are combined in Figure 5.1 which shows that most of those who walked lived within ten minutes of the health centre, and that buses were the main form of transport for longer journeys.

There have been plans to increase the number of health centres in Glasgow, but there are difficulties in locating these because of the mobility of the population and the fact that general practitioners may have patients scattered over a wide area. One method has been to develop computer programmes which take into account population projections and access to bus routes.(14) However, the cost of bus fares from peripheral housing estates in Glasgow is considerable, especially for mothers with young children, and may be a disincentive to seeking medical advice. The alternative might be to leave the health centre, as illustrated by the following interviewer's comment:

9-year-old daughter of a lorry driver: 'Parents had no complaint about doctor, but length of journey, then poor appointment system is making them consider transferring to a nearer doctor.

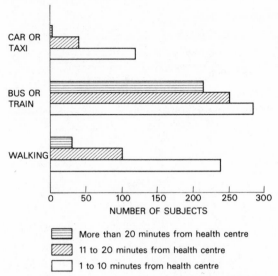

NUMBER OF SUBJECTS

▭ More than 20 minutes from health centre
▨ 11 to 20 minutes from health centre
▢ 1 to 10 minutes from health centre

FIGURE 5.1   Method of travel and time to health centre

In the present survey those who had a long walk or bus journey
to the health centre had significantly higher incongruous medical
lay referral scores.   Studies from America have related distance to
the utilization of medical care,(15,16) and one study in the United
Kingdom found that the size of practice lists was the main factor
in determining how far patients had to travel.(17)   The fact that
the medical symptom 'iceberg' was related to long patient journeys
in the present survey raises questions about the size of health
centres in conurbations such as Glasgow.   The problems of siting
health centres in conurbations with high population mobility are
discussed in the chapter on implications, but in general the larger
a health centre the more dispersed will be the patients registered
there.   This may not affect those with private transport, but those
without a car are placed at a distinct disadvantage, particularly
the elderly and mothers with young families.   These vulnerable
groups are the least able to undertake long walks, especially if
unwell and in bad weather.   They are also those most likely to be
put off by the cost of public transport.   There would seem to be a
strong case for more consideration being given to patient access,
rather than to the presumed economies of size, when planning primary
care facilities.   In addition, when health centres reach a certain
size the management problems increase considerably, with the need
for more administrative staff.

DOCTORS AND THE HEALTH CENTRE

When asked about their previous experience of doctors and hospitals,
the majority of responses were rated as favourable, as indicated in
Figure 5.2, but about 6 per cent of the answers were definitely
unfavourable.   This small group tended to have more symptoms than
others and also to refer more trivia, which suggests that previous

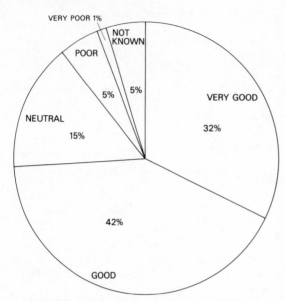

FIGURE 5.2   Previous experience of doctors and hospitals
             (1,344 subjects)

experience of doctors and hospitals may have been the result of
referral behaviour rather than the other way round.   Consumer
assessments of medical care, however, present problems of reactivity
in that the subjects know they are also being evaluated.(18)   There
was in fact considerable interviewer variation in the responses
elicited to this open-ended question.

   In general, people were favourably impressed by their contacts
with doctors as illustrated by the following comments:

54-year-old housewife: 'Struck by attention she got from general
practitioner after twenty years of no contact, and by personal touch
in National Health Service which she thought had died out.'

89-year-old widow: 'Very appreciative of help and attention obtained
from general practitioner.'

Others were less happy with their doctors, sometimes for specific
reasons such as the following:

62-year-old housewife: 'Felt inhibited with male doctors - "If I
had a lady doctor, I could go down to talk to her differently" -
complained several times of embarrassment when having the smear
test.'

   Figure 5.3 shows that over half those interviewed preferred to
see their own doctor, and almost three-quarters would have wanted
to see at least one of the practice, when asked whom they would like
to see first if wishing to consult a doctor.   The fact that patients
have a marked preference for seeing their own doctor has been confirmed by other surveys in the United Kingdom (13,19) and also in
Australia.(20)   An intriguing study from Poland reported that the

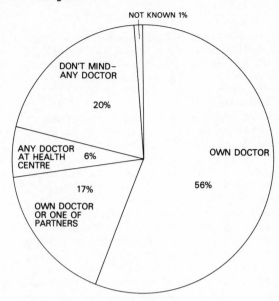

FIGURE 5.3   Preference for doctor of first contact (1,344 subjects)

majority of those interviewed would like to have been able to choose
their own doctor.(21)   The concept of a personal family doctor is
therefore by no means a thing of the past.   In the present survey,
preference for one's own doctor was associated with an increased
tendency to seek medical advice.

The number of subjects who said they preferred the health centre
to their doctor's previous surgery was 70 per cent, and only 10 per
cent expressed a preference for the latter.   But as the interviewing
started within a year of the health centre opening, several people
had not yet been there.   When asked if they thought the health
centre arrangements could be improved in any way, most people had
no comments to make, but 37 per cent had some criticisms, of which
the majority (22 per cent) concerned the appointments system.   The
main difficulty seemed to be delays in getting appointments, or
occasionally being turned away.   There were also almost a hundred
respondents who complained about being kept waiting when they came
at the time given them for an appointment.

Many subjects, however, welcomed the health centre and also the
appointments system, as illustrated by the following comment:

34-year-old accountant: 'Feels that the health centre is a great
improvement, and because of the appointments system, the general
practitioner has more time to spend with his patient.'

Others reacted less favourably, as for instance, the following:

49-year-old tailoress: 'Health Centre too clinical - no friendly
atmosphere - felt more like a number than a human being.   Too
impersonal - you feel you're just a nuisance to them.'

There were several other specific comments, but none of them
were made by more than 2 per cent of those interviewed.   But 22

respondents criticized the receptionists, who were seen as a barrier between the patient and their doctor with whom there was a lack of personal contact. One study of the way in which receptionists balanced the demands of doctors and patients concluded that on the whole they did so without abusing their power.(22)   In all, 19 people said that they had no choice of doctor, or could not see their own doctor, or saw different doctors each time, with the additional comment from a few that notes were not kept up to date; 18 subjects said that they thought the health centre was impersonal, and the same number that the surgery hours were inconvenient. The lack of a surgery in the evening or on Saturday mornings was part-icularly resented by those who found it difficult to get time off work. Criticisms of the physical amenities at the health centre were made by 14 respondents, and the same number complained about difficulties in getting prescriptions or sickness certificates. A further 13 people criticized the doctors for being too hurried or impersonal, and the same number complained about delays in getting home visits. Lastly, 10 subjects each criticized the emergency service and the lack of privacy in the reception area. The recep-tion area is an important part of a health centre (23) and an open-plan design makes it very difficult for receptionists to carry on a private conversation or telephone calls with patients.

The acceptability of changing to a health centre depends on what had gone before, and at least some of the practices had well-run surgeries in good premises. Also, those who made criticisms or suggested improvements tended to have more mental and social symptoms. However, the need for more information about patients' attitudes to health centres has been stressed in a recent review, (24) although in the same source it was stated that patients were well satisfied and had few complaints. In a sense this was true because the majority were pleased with the health centre, and criticisms were not necessarily voiced as complaints. On the whole most people are tolerant of shortcomings in public services, and tend not to be critical unless specifically asked. There is there-fore a tacit lack of communication between professional providers and the recipients of care, which may be particularly true for the less well-educated.(25)

Other studies in the United Kingdom support the impression that patients prefer new health centres, but that the introduction of an appointments system is the main cause of dissatisfaction.(26,27) The majority of general practitioners in Britain have appointments of some kind,(28) and patients appear to get used to this in spite of initial criticisms.(29) One review of the literature (5) con-cluded that conflicting findings about attitudes towards appoint-ments systems could be explained by the fact that people tend to prefer the status quo to which they are accustomed. The introduc-tion of an appointments system in a London general practice (30) was found to shift demand away from the young towards the old and mentally ill who tend to be part of the symptom 'iceberg'.

The impression as recorded by one interviewer was of general approval of the facilities provided by the health centre, with the common complain that one cannot be ill by appointment. The follow-ing are some comments about the appointments system which illustrate a fairly widespread concern:

42-year-old wife of academic: 'Cannot get appointment when want it. May wait for two days for a child - so doctor has to call.'

30-year-old unemployed storeman: 'If phone for appointment when ill, and appointment given for several days ahead, then patients just ask for a house call, which puts more load on doctor.'

44-year-old taxi-driver: 'According to this man many people use the hospital outpatients because of delay or difficulty in getting appointments at the health centre.'

4-year-old girl: 'Mother said difficult to get appointment - delay especially bad for children.'

2-year-old daughter of a window cleaner: 'Mother's main grouse about the health centre was seldom seeing own doctor - this had come with the appointments system.'

However, not all comments were complaints, and some welcomed the appointments system, for instance.

22-year-old housewife: 'Thought health centre and appointments excellent. Rather than call out emergency doctors, would go to casualty department - this fairer on general practitioner.'

MEDICINE TAKING

The number of subjects taking prescribed and unprescribed medicines is indicated in Figure 5.4. About one-third of those interviewed were taking prescribed medicines and just over a third of these were repeat prescriptions, with a small number of people taking medicines prescribed for someone else. A similar proportion were taking unpre-scribed medicines, mainly bought from a chemist. Almost all those obtained from another source were from a newsagent or corner shop.

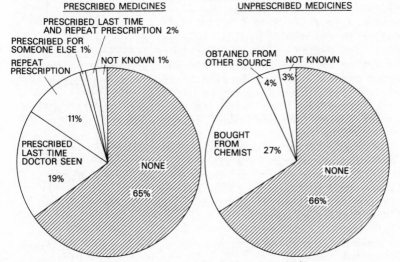

FIGURE 5.4 Medicine taking (1,344 subjects)

Although the numbers of people taking prescribed and unprescribed
medicines were very much the same, more prescribed medicines were
being used than unprescribed because there were more individuals
taking several prescribed medicines at one time, as shown by Figure
5.5.

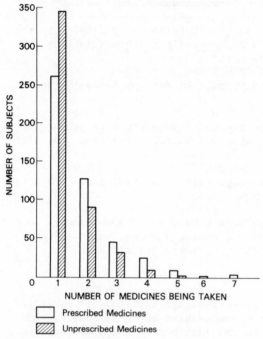

FIGURE 5.5   Numbers of medicines taken

Compared with other studies from the United Kingdom,(31,32,33)
these findings suggest that fewer people in Glasgow were taking
unprescribed medicines, both overall and in relation to prescribed
medicines.   The results are more comparable to those reported from
a survey in France,(34) and similar to a study in Canada,(35)
although the latter did not distinguish between prescribed and
unprescribed medicines.   However, in a survey in Australia, two-
thirds of the sample had taken some form of medicine in the previous
two weeks.(8)   Considerable variations in prescribing habits have
been noted at both national (36) and regional levels,(37) as well
as between groups of general practitioners (38) and within one area
for a particular medicine.(39)

The actual prescribed and unprescribed medicines being taken are
shown in Table 5.4.   Compound medicines were classified according
to the main ingredient.   The commonest prescribed medicines were
sedatives and tranquillizers, followed by skin preparations; and
the commonest unprescribed medicines were antipyretics and analgesics.   Antipyretics were by far the most frequently used medicines
and included aspirin and aspirin mixtures like Beecham's powders,
as well as anti-inflammatory agents such as Indocid.   Most antipyretics were not prescribed and many were in the form of Askit
powders, a local mixture of aspirin and caffeine.   Sedatives,

TABLE 5.4 Types of medicines being taken (1,344 subjects)

Types of medicine	Number of subjects taking medicines (%)	
	Prescribed	Unprescribed
Antipyretics	23 (2%)	221 (16%)
Antibiotics	48 (4%)	1 (<1%)
Analgesics	53 (4%)	64 (5%)
Sedatives and tranquillizers	59 (4%)	0 -
Hypnotics	51 (4%)	1 (<1%)
Antidepressants	10 (1%)	0 -
Anticonvulsants	8 (1%)	1 (<1%)
Other central nervous system	5 (<1%)	0 -
Cough	53 (4%)	53 (4%)
Upper respiratory	18 (1%)	27 (2%)
Lower respiratory	38 (3%)	6 (<1%)
Antacids	33 (3%)	45 (3%)
Laxatives	5 (<1%)	47 (4%)
Other alimentary system	11 (1%)	11 (1%)
Iron	49 (4%)	7 (1%)
Other minerals	8 (1%)	3 (<1%)
Vitamins	16 (1%)	45 (3%)
Systemic hormones	23 (2%)	0 -
Other nutrition and metabolism	11 (1%)	4 (<1%)
Skin	54 (4%)	39 (3%)
Hair	2 (<1%)	13 (1%)
Heart	40 (3%)	1 (<1%)
Circulation	32 (2%)	1 (<1%)
Diuretics	14 (1%)	0 -
Other urinary system	16 (1%)	1 (<1%)
Contraceptive pill	4 (<1%)	0 -
Other gynaecological system	2 (<1%)	2 (<1%)
Eyes	10 (1%)	5 (<1%)
Ears	7 (1%)	5 (<1%)
Counter-irritants	8 (1%)	10 (1%)
Allergies	11 (1%)	0 -
Other medicines	3 (<1%)	11 (1%)
Unidentified medicines	44 (3%)	9 (1%)
Other treatments	2 (<1%)	2 (<1%)

tranquillizers and hypnotics were almost exclusively prescribed.
Analgesics, cough medicines, and skin preparations were obtained
both with and without prescription, and reflected the prevalence
of the common symptom groups.

In general, other studies of medicine taking in the United
Kingdom confirm the preponderance of analgesics and antipyretics,
skin preparations, cough medicines and medicines acting on the
alimentary tract.(32) However, there were some striking differences
from another British survey,(33) which reported, for instance, that
only 10 per cent of skin preparations were prescribed, whereas 59
per cent of such preparations were prescribed in Glasgow. Several

studies have confirmed the importance of psychotropic drugs,(40,41) the use of which has risen dramatically over the past few years,(42) especially for tranquillizers.

The striking thing about the unprescribed medicines in the present study was the importance of antipyretics, which comprised 35 per cent of unprescribed medicines, and with analgesics accounted for 45 per cent of all unprescribed medicines. This is a much higher proportion than that found in the British survey referred to above,(33) and was at least partly due to the use of local compound analgesics which have been related to the incidence of renal disease in the west of Scotland.(43,44)

The taking of both prescribed and unprescribed medicines tended to increase with the number of symptoms, and with people's tendency to refer medical symptoms professional whether for 'trivia' or not. Interestingly, those who were part of the medical symptom 'iceberg' took significantly less of both prescribed and unprescribed medicines.

Interviewers' comments indicated that some people had definite views on self-medication, which was sometimes cheaper because of prescription charges, as indicated by the following quotations:

63-year-old school cleaner: 'Quite keen on self-medication - "I doctor myself" - and especially on camphorated oil as a cure-all; also mentioned cod-liver oil. Seemed to have a detailed catalogue of do's and don'ts and medicines to use and avoid.'

17-year-old shop assistant: 'Worked in chemist and bought medicines for minor complaints. Thought many did the same since prescription charges sometimes levelled the score.'

Other comments mentioned more bizarre remedies such as the 68-year-old widow who hung up cut onions to draw diseases, and the 59-year-old housewife whose ear trouble started when her husband poured whisky into her ear.

In addition to questions on medicine taking, a simple medical knowledge test was asked, as well as questions on whether people would go straight to a doctor if in doubt about a symptom, and whether they thought home remedies were as good as prescribed medicines. Most of those interviewed did not think that home remedies were as good as prescribed medicines, and would have gone straight to a doctor if in doubt about a symptom. Neither of these simple attitudinal questions, nor the medical knowledge score, gave significant correlations with the main dependent variables for symptom prevalence or referral behaviour. There have been several studies based on the assessment of attitudes towards health and medical services, but these tend to be tautologous, without always adding very much to our understanding of what is happening.

FAMILY PLANNING

Those who were married and of child-bearing age, whether answering for themselves or a child, were asked about family planning. Figures 5.6 and 5.7 show the results for the methods of contraception used and for the sources of advice and supplies. Of those who

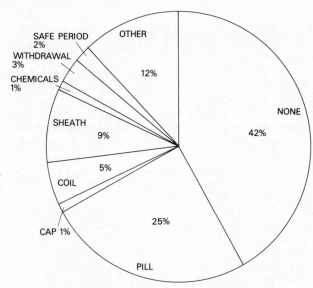

(Percentage out of 602 respondents who were married
and of child-bearing age, whether being interviewed
about themselves or a child)

FIGURE 5.6   Methods of contraception used

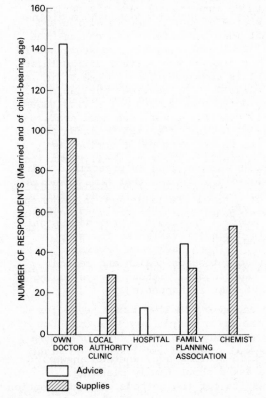

FIGURE 5.7   Sources of contraceptive advice and supplies

replied almost half used no contraception at all, and of those who
did the majority were on the pill. Almost all those classified as
'other' had been sterilized, mainly the wife, with or without a
hysterectomy, but often the husband by vasectomy. The main source
of advice and supplies was the family doctor, followed by the Family
Planning Association clinic for advice, and the chemist without a
prescription for supplies. The majority (85 per cent) of those who
answered thought that facilities for obtaining family planning
advice and contraceptive supplies were adequate. Of those who did
not, most felt that there should be more publicity, and some commented that there could have been better advice from doctors. Others
thought there should have been more family planning clinics, but very
few suggested that these services should be free.

These findings confirm the shift towards the pill as a method of
contraception, which has been reported by other studies in the
United Kingdom,(45,46,47,48) as well as in other countries such as
America,(49) Australia (5) and Belgium.(51) There may, however, be
considerable regional variations in the use of oral contraception,
(52) and one survey in America reported a decline in recent years.
(53) Of those answering as being married and of child-bearing age
12 per cent had been sterilized, which appears to be on the increase
as a means of curtailing family size.(54,55) There were 5 per cent
replying in the present survey who used traditional non-medical
methods of birth control, which are still of importance.(56,57)

Less than a quarter of all those interviewed gave any definite
answer to questions about the source of contraceptive advice and
supplies. It is surprising that more respondents did not use the
Family Planning Association or local authority clinics where contraceptive supplies were free at the time of the survey, unlike those
obtained from family doctors. This adds substance to the criticisms
about more publicity being required for the services available.

The important part played by doctors as sources of advice about
family planning, especially oral contraceptives, has been confirmed
by other studies from Britain,(58) Denmark (59) and Holland.(60)
Most general practitioners in the United Kingdom prescribe the
pill,(61) but only a few offer a complete range of family planning
services.(62) Surveys in Australia indicate that the majority of
women would prefer to consult their own doctor about family planning,
(63) but that only a minority of general practitioners initiate such
discussions.(64) There is now evidence that the medical profession
is reacting to these demands by actually teaching medical students
and doctors about family planning.(65)

The following interviewer's comments illustrate some of the
anxieties felt about family planning largely due to lack of confidence and communication.

3-year-old daughter of heating engineer: 'Mother meant to go for
family planning but "feart of the pill; people say it's O.K. but
I'm feart" - Would like family planning advice but not sure where
to go. Doesn't want to ask general practitioner because he might
prescribe the pill without examination and she is afraid of this.'

8-year-old son of auxiliary nurse: 'Mother has asked own doctor for
the pill and literature about this method of contraception but has

never received any help or advice. Not enough reliable information available about the pill except what one reads in the newspapers. One reads of doubts about the pill and there is nobody ready to talk and give assurance.'

3-year-old son of a printer: 'Mother pleasant and intelligent with four children. Never knew about safe period until recently asked general practitioner after priest had said it was all right.'

These extracts highlight the difficulties of a minority, but it was found that those who used no contraception at all and went nowhere for advice or supplies were more likely to be part of the medical symptom 'iceberg'. Subjects who had been sterilized had significantly more behavioural problems with children and social symptoms, and together with those on the pill were more likely to seek medical advice.

REFERENCES

1   Marsh, G.N. and McNay, R.A. (1974), Team Work Load in an English General Practice, 'British Medical Journal', 1/5903, 315-18.
2   Bain, D.J.G. (1975), Health Centre Practice in Livingstone New Town, 'Health Bulletin', 31/6, 290-6.
3   Office of Health Economics (1968), 'General Practice Today', London.
4   Fry, J. (1972), Twenty-one Years of General Practice, 'Journal of the Royal College of General Practitioners', 22/131, 521-8.
5   Office of Health Economics (1974), 'The Work of Primary Medical Care', London.
6   'Journal of the Royal College of General Practitioners' (1973), Patterns of Work, Report 16, 16-23.
7   Wilder, C.S. (1972), Physician Visits - Volume and Interval since Last Visit - U.S. 1969, 'Vital Health Statistics', 10/72.
8   Bridges-Webb, C. (1974), The Traralgon Health & Illness Survey: Prevalence of Illness and Use of Health Care, 'International Journal of Epidemiology', 3, 37-46.
9   Oliemans, A.P. and De Waard, F. (1970), Morbidity in General Practice, 'Huisarts Wetensch', 13/1, 24-8.
10 Office of Population Censuses and Surveys (1973), 'The General Household Survey', HMSO, London.
11 Greenlick, M.R. et al. (1973), Role of Telephone in Total Medical Care, 'Medical Care', 11/2, 121-34.
12 Pope, C.R. et al. (1971), Use of Telephone for Reporting Symptoms, 'Journal of Health and Social Behaviour', 12/2, 155-62.
13 Millar, D.G. (1972), Health Centres and Excellent Medicine - A Patient Survey, 'Journal of the Royal College of General Practitioners', 22, 866-74.
14 Robertson, I.M.F. (1974), Personal communication.
15 Weiss, J.E. and Greenlick, M.R. (1970), Determinants of Medical Care Utilization, 'Medical Care', 8/6, 456-62.
16 Brooks, C.M. (1973), Associations among Distance, Patient Satis-faction, and Utilization of Two Types of Inter-city Clinics, 'Medical Care', 11, 373-83.

17   Pinsent, R.J.F.H. and Peacock, J.B. (1973), Going to the Doctor, 'Journal of the Royal College of General Practitioners', 23/131, 404-10.

18   Lebow, J.C. (1974), Consumer Assessments of the Quality of Medical Care, 'Medical Care', 12, 328-37.

19   Kaim-Caudle, P.R. and Marsh, G.N. (1975), Patient Satisfaction Survey in General Practice, 'British Medical Journal', 5952, 262-4.

20   Watson, D.S. (1971), Consumer Demand for Health Services, 'Medical Journal of Australia', 2, 147-52.

21   Bejnarowicz, J. and Ostrowska, A. (1972), Opinions of Polish Urban Population about the Health System, 'Paper at 3rd International Conference of Social Science and Medicine - Elsinore'.

22   Lubin, M. (1972), Power of the Receptionists: Myth or Reality? Unpublished paper, Bedford College, London.

23   Butler, N.K. (1972), The Reception Area, 'Update', 5/7, 725-34.

24   British Health Care and Technology (1974), 'Health Centres', Health and Social Services Journal, London.

25   Rossenblatt, A. et al. (1970), Help Seeking for Family Problems: a Survey of Utilization and Satisfaction, 'American Journal of Psychiatry', 128, 1136-40.

26   Woods, J.O. et al. (1974), Health Centre Assessment by Patients, 'Journal of the Royal College of General Practitioners', 24/138, 23-7.

27   Patterson, J.S. (1975), Patients' Attitudes to Health Centres, 'Health Bulletin', 33/2, 52-7.

28   Irvine, D. and Jefferys, M. (1971), B.M.A. Planning Unit Survey of General Practice, 'British Medical Journal', 4, 535-43.

29   Bevan, J.M. and Draper, G.J. (1967), 'Appointment Systems in General Practice', Oxford University Press, London.

30   Morrell, D.C. and Kasap, H.S. (1972), Effect of Appointments System on Demand for Medical Care, 'International Journal of Epidemiology', 1/2, 143-51.

31   Jefferys, M. et al. (1960), Consumption of Medicines on a Working Class Housing Estate, 'British Journal of Social and Preventive Medicine', 14, 64-76.

32   Wadsworth, M.E.J., Butterfield, W.J.H. and Blaney, R. (1971), 'Health and Sickness: The Choice of Treatment', Tavistock, London.

33   Dunnell, K. and Cartwright, A. (1972), 'Medicine Takers, Prescribers and Hoarders', Routledge & Kegan Paul, London.

34   Guillot, C. et al. (1971), Morbidity in a Given Population and Its Connection with the Use of Medical Services, 'Rev. Epid. Med. Soc.', 19/4, 311-51.

35   Vobecky, J. et al. (1972), Population Health Care Practices; an Epidemiological Study, 'Canadian Journal of Public Health', 63/4, 304-10.

36   Dunlop, D. and Inch, R.S. (1972), Variations in European Medical and Pharmaceutical Practice, 'British Medical Journal', 3/5829, 749-52.

37   Martin, J.P. (1957), 'Social Aspects of Prescribing', Heinemann, London.

38   Joyce, C.R.B. et al. (1967), Personal Factors as a Cause of Differences in Prescribing by General Practitioners, 'British Journal of Preventive and Social Medicine', 21, 170-7.

39 Wade, O.L. and Hood, H.E. (1972), An Analysis of Prescribing an
    Hypnotic in the Community, 'British Journal of Preventive and
    Social Medicine', 26, 121-8.
40 Patterson, J.S. (1972), How Many Drugs do I Use?, 'Journal of
    the Royal College of General Practitioners', 22/116, 191-4.
41 Jenner, G.G. (1973), Prescriptions in General Practice, 'New
    Zealand Medical Journal', 79/500, 296-9.
42 Office of Health Economics (1972), 'Medicine and Society', London.
43 Murray, R.M. (1972), Analgesic Nephropathy: Removal of Phenac-
    etin from Proprietary Analgesics, 'British Medical Journal',
    5833, 131-2.
44 Murray, R.M. (1973), The Geographic Distribution of Analgesic
    Nephropathy, 'Health Bulletin', 31/1, 32.
45 Langford, C.M. (1969), Birth Control Practice in Britain,
    'Family Planning', 17/4, 89-92.
46 Cartwright, A. (1970), 'Parents and Family Planning Services',
    Routledge & Kegan Paul, London.
47 Cartwright, A. (1974), Inadequacies of Contraceptive Services
    in England and Wales, 'Journal of Reproduction and Fertility',
    37, 459-65.
48 Clarke, M. (1972), Use of F.P.A. Clinics in a London Borough,
    'Journal of Biosocial Science', 4/3, 325-32.
49 Pomeroy, R. et al. (1972), Family Planning Practices of Low
    Income Women in Two Communities, 'American Journal of Public
    Health', 62, 1123-9.
50 Wood, C. (1974), A Study of Attitudes to Contraceptives in a
    Middle Class Group of Women, 'Medical Journal of Australia',
    1, 659-60.
51 Cliquet, R.L. (1972), Knowledge, Practice and Effectiveness of
    Contraception in Belgium, 'Journal of Biosocial Science', 4/1,
    41-73.
52 Larsson, C.V. and Trost, J. (1970), Consumption of Contraceptive
    Pills in Sweden in 1969, 'Lakartidningen', 67, 85-90.
53 Bouvier, L.F. (1973), Changes in the Use of Oral Contraceptives,
    'Social Biology', 20/1, 51-63.
54 Presser, H.B. and Bumpass, L.L. (1972), Acceptability of Contra-
    ceptive Sterilisation among U.S. Couples 1970, 'Family Planning
    Perspectives', 4/4, 18-26.
55 Siegal, E. et al. (1973), Family Planning - Changing Attitudes
    and Practices among Low Income Women between 1967 and 1970/71,
    'American Journal of Public Health', 63, 255-61.
56 Glatthaar, E. (1970), Traditional Contraceptive Methods, 'Ther.
    Umsch.', 27/10, 646-51.
57 Harvey, P.D. (1973), Non-Medical Birth Control, 'American
    Journal of Public Health', 63, 473-5.
58 Donaldson, P.J. (1970), Physicians and Methods of Birth
    Planning, 'Rhode Island Medical Journal', 53/8, 419-23.
59 Backer, P. and Sele, V. (1970), Contraception in General
    Practice, 'Ugeskr. Laeg.', 132/5, 227-31.
60 Moors, J.P.C. (1970), Family Planning, 'Thesis', Utrecht.
61 Gillie, I.M.S. and Ludkin, S. (1971), General Practice Family
    Planning Services in Co. Durham, 'Medical Officer', 125/24,
    305-7.

62 Brennan, M.E. and Opit, L.J. (1974), Extension of Family
    Planning Service in General Practice, 'British Medical Journal',
    2, 30-3.
63 Berry, G. et al. (1972), Survey on Attitudes to Family Planning
    among 360 Brisbane Women, 'Medical Journal of Australia', 2/15,
    820-6.
64 Barson, M. and Wood, C. (1972), The Role of the General Prac-
    titioner in Family Planning, 'Medical Journal of Australia',
    1/21, 1069-71.
65 Barley, N.H. (1973), Family Planning Clinic in General Practice,
    'Journal of the Royal College of General Practitioners',
    23/134, 663-4.

Chapter 6

USE AND PERCEPTION
OF SOCIAL WORK

'As yet we know remarkably little about the effectiveness of our
welfare and social work services.'
          (Social Work Scotland - Report of a Working Party - 1969)

Medical and social symptoms are inevitably interwoven, and so is the
manner of their referral. A comparatively recent point of primary
referral in Scotland are social work departments, and it is therefore important to look at their use when considering symptoms and
referral in the community. Such use will be reflected by the amount
of contact with social workers, which will depend on people's knowledge of what social workers do and how to gain access to them. It
is also relevant to see if there are other sources of assistance
available in the community.

CONTACT WITH SOCIAL WORK

Only 9 per cent of those interviewed had seen a social worker during
the past year, and only 14 per cent said that they knew someone else
who had been to a social worker - mainly friends and acquaintances
rather than relatives. Figure 6.1 indicates the reasons for seeing
a social worker, both for respondents themselves and for others
whom they knew. Only one or two people made inappropriate referrals
such as for antenatal care or employment. The commonest reasons
for subjects themselves contacting a social worker related to
children, whereas acquaintances who had been to social workers were
said to have gone mainly about adult relationships or illness,
which was perhaps not surprising. It is interesting that problems
such as marital difficulties and crime, which might involve personal stigma were mentioned more often for others seeing social
workers than for respondents themselves. In general fewer social
work contacts were made because of the elderly than for problems of
adults, children or financial difficulties.
    There appears to have been comparatively little research into
the functioning of social work in the United Kingdom, and the need
for social workers to define their aims, roles, and methods, within

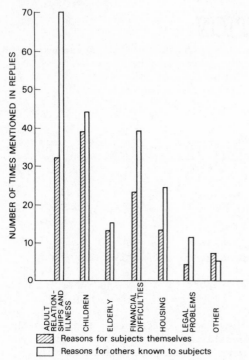

FIGURE 6.1   Reasons for seeing a social worker

some analytical framework has been stressed.(1)   The importance of
cooperation between social work and primary medical care has been
frequently emphasized in view of the extensive overlap between
these two areas of concern.(2,3,4,5)   One study from America (6)
found that those with a higher occupational and educational status
tended to use social workers more, and another from England (7)
reported that the majority of problems brought by social work
clients concerned the elderly and disabled, in contrast to the
findings from the present survey.

For those who had been in contact with social workers, reactions
varied as illustrated by the following interviewer's comments:

57-year-old housewife: 'Can not speak highly enough of medical
social worker in hospital. Her husband was unemployed due to ill
health and they were desperately worried that they wouldn't be able
to pay rent, which they find very high. Social worker obtained
help from some fund, and husband obtained employment two weeks ago,
so that worry is over.'

62-year-old unemployed labourer: 'Subject and wife foster two
children, one of whom causes some anxiety. Wife doesn't keep very
well. She had two operations on her jaw, with removal of bone.
She was rather concerned that she got so little help and support
from the present social worker who has only visited her once despite
repeated phone calls.'

KNOWLEDGE OF SOCIAL WORK

Figure 6.2 indicates the range of answers given when respondents
were asked what sort of problems they thought social workers dealt
with. The results are shown as proportions of the number of times
items were mentioned in replies, which often included several problems relevant to social work. About a third of those asked seemed

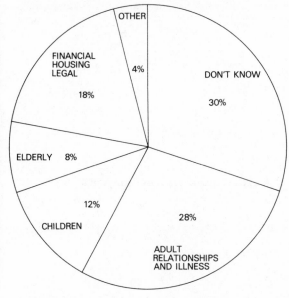

FIGURE 6.2 Problems
dealt with by social
workers (1,772 items
mentioned)

to have no idea what social workers did, and the problems most
frequently mentioned concerned personal relationships amongst
adults, followed by financial difficulties and children. The
elderly did not figure so prominently either in the perceived or
actual reasons for social work referral. Although the numbers
involved in the actual referrals shown in Figure 6.1 are much
smaller than the answers given in Figure 6.2, it seems that people
perceived social work as being mainly concerned with family and
domestic difficulties involving adults, whereas in practice it was
the more specific problems of children that were more likely to be
referred.

When asked how they would contact a social worker, about half
the respondents did not know, and almost as many would have gone
to the health centre as would have contacted a social work department, as indicated by Figure 6.3. Only 20 per cent knew the location of the nearest social work department, the commonest incorrect
reply being the health centre; but, as shown in Figure 6.4, the
majority simply said that they didn't know where the social work
department was located. In fact at the time of the survey, only a
quarter of the practices at the health centre had an attached
social worker. Similar results were found in a study in England
(7) where half the referrals to one social work department were
initiated by a third partly mainly from a health service, and the
great majority of clients had not known where the social work

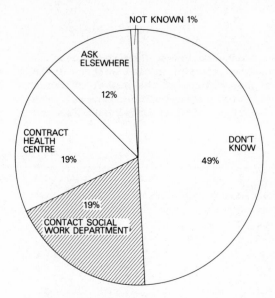

FIGURE 6.3 How to contact a social worker (1,344 subjects)

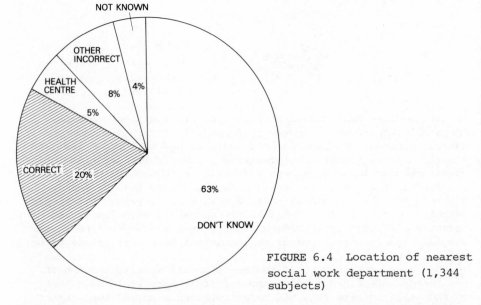

FIGURE 6.4 Location of nearest
social work department (1,344
subjects)

department was. In the present survey, those answering for children
were more likely than other adults to know how to contact a social
worker, and also to know the whereabouts of the nearest social work
department.

People's perceptions of social work were varied and often did
not reflect the professional image of social workers themselves, as
illustrated by the following interviewers' comments:

40-year-old wife of machine operator: 'Open and cooperative; seven
children but house quite tidy. Parting shot on social workers when

their function was briefly explained - "that's something you'd try
and deal with yourself, you wouldn't think of asking anyone for
help".'

55-year-old school janitor: 'Talked fairly coherently about social
problems. Thought social workers were flogging a dead horse, though
well-intentioned, because root problem with children and youths
was parents.'

12-year-old daughter of unemployed lorry driver: 'Family obviously
hard up. Not very clean though the house was tidy. Mother having
psychiatric trouble and father off work as injured in an accident.
Thinks it very unlikely that firm will take him back. When wife
lost her purse the social security would only give them a £2 food
voucher. They were absolutely desperate with six children, and
went to "The Welfare - it's the place where you go when you are
absolutely at rock bottom, you know it's connected with the cruelty
people". (Address mentioned was of social work department.)'

The picture of people's perceptions of social work which emerges
from these results hardly fulfils the promise of the Social Work
(Scotland) Act of 1968,(8) which stated - 'it shall be the duty of
every local authority to promite social welfare by making available
advice, guidance and assistance on such a scale as may be appropriate for their area.' In view of the social problems of Glasgow
it is difficult to imagine what might be an appropriate scale. A
report of a working party on the Social Work (Scotland) Act (9)
thought that 'Undoubtedly the social work department, when it
becomes well known, will be used as a general advice bureau and
point of access...'. With supplies of staff being inevitably
limited, perhaps it is just as well that social work departments
have not fulfilled these admirable ideals.
    One of the problems of social work is the breadth of its remit,
which is stated in very general terms. Inevitably it is defined
in different ways by different people with the result that there are
conflicting expectations,(10) and also difficulties of demarcation
in that social work spills over into almost every social service
including health. Some have criticized social work as being an
agent of social control,(11) and others have condemned the tendency
to confuse economic difficulties with personal failure and the
arrogance of not accepting practical problems, but always looking
for underlying causes.(12) Several writers have emphasized the
need for criteria and goals in social casework,(13) and the
importance of research models for evaluating social work.(14)
    The fact that social work clearly impinges on medical care opens
up possibilities for both cooperation and conflict. In some areas
in the United Kingdom many practices have an attached social
worker,(15) whose importance for family psychiatry has been stressed
in several countries.(16,17,18,19) However, the advent of social
work departments has created anxiety amongst some family doctors,
(20) and concern about the deployment of existing medical social
workers in Britain.(21)
    The findings from the present survey suggest that people were
just as likely to perceive the health centre as a source of social

work advice as they were a social work department. The extent to
which social problems are referred to family doctors has been well
documented,(22) although there is evidence that some doctors are
unaware or resentful of this role.(23) In view of the fact that
general practitioners are a well-known source of referral with whom
everyone in the United Kingdom should be registered, it would seem
sensible to build on this system, by attaching social workers to
existing practices rather than setting up completely new departments.
This should become increasingly feasible with the growing numbers of
group practices and health centres in Britain, and the tendency for
a team approach to primary medical care.(24)

OTHER SOURCES OF ASSISTANCE

Respondents were asked whether they had had any contacts with other
helping agencies during the past twelve months, and if so why. As
shown by Table 6.1, about 22 per cent of those interviewed had had
contact with other helping agencies apart from doctors or social

TABLE 6.1   Other helping agencies

Other helping agencies contacted in the past twelve months	Number of subjects (%)
Not known	23 (2%)
None	1023 (76%)
Health Visitor	62 (5%)
District nurse or midwife	60 (5%)
Hospital Nurse	31 (2%)
Home help	18 (1%)
Child guidance	17 (1%)
School clinic	10 (1%)
Antenatal or baby clinic	9 (1%)
Other clinic or helping agency	32 (2%)
Multiple helping agencies	59 (4%)
Total	1344 (100%)

workers. Over half these contacts had been with members of the
nursing profession, either as health visitors, district nurses,
midwives, or in hospital. Following these came home helps, child
guidance, and school doctors or clinics. The main reasons for such
contacts were physical illness (dressings, injections, etc.), and
child welfare or a new baby. These were followed by mental illness
or behavioural disorders, and problems with the elderly. Such
requirements correspond to the predominance of nurses as the main
helping agents apart from doctors and social workers.

The majority of health visitors and home nurses now work in association with family doctors in the United Kingdom, and a high proportion of practices have some kind of nursing attachment.(2) Nurses are therefore an important part of the health care team,(25, 26) and there have been several evaluations of these attachments all indicating the success of such schemes.(27,28,29,30)   There are however considerable variations in the way in which the skills of attached nurses are used,(31) and many nurses working in the community in Scotland have combined the roles of home nursing, midwifery, and health visiting.(32)   The respective functions of nurses and social workers in the community are not always as clearly defined as might be expected, especially for health visitors in Britain.   One study in America (6) found that nurses and social workers were complementary in that the higher socio-economic groups tended to go to social workers, with the lower socio-economic groups preferring nurses.

Respondents were also asked if there was anyone in their neighbourhood to whom lots of people from round about went for advice about problems.   The results are shown in Table 6.2.   Only 16 per cent said there was anyone in the neighbourhood to whom people went with problems.   Interestingly the commonest perceived sources of such advice were the respondents themselves, followed by friends or

TABLE 6.2   Sources of neighbourhood advice

Source of neighbourhood advice	Number of subjects (%)
Not known	146 (11%)
None	983 (73%)
Self	51 (4%)
Spouse	17 (1%)
Parent	15 (1%)
Other relatives	15 (1%)
Friend or neighbour	41 (3%)
Other informal individuals	8 (0.5%)
Councillor	19 (2%)
Minister or priest	10 (0.5%)
Other formal individuals	13 (1%)
Tenants' association	7 (0.5%)
Other organization	7 (0.5%)
Combination of sources	11 (1%)
Total	1344 (100%)

neighbours.   Local authority councillors and then ministers or
priests were the most frequently mentioned formal sources of advice.
The only individual to be named was one particular local councillor,
who was named several times.   The commonest organizations acting as
sources of advice were tenants' associations.   No doctors or social
workers were mentioned, perhaps because such professionals tend not
to live in the same areas as their patients or clients in central
Glasgow.   These findings hardly suggest a flourishing 'lay referral
system' or active community self-help.

The use of other helping agencies increased for those with higher
symptom frequencies, mainly because of nursing care due to illness.
Respondents who mentioned informal individuals as sources of neighbourhood advice had significantly more children's behavioural
symptoms and also social symptoms.

REFERENCES

1 Burton, J.W. (1973), Contending Approaches to Social Work,
   'Social Work Today', 4/17, 528-30.
2 Office of Health Economics (1974), 'The Work of Primary
   Medical Care', London.
3 MacLean, U. (1973), Interface between Medicine and Social Work,
   Public and Professional Attitudes, 'British Journal of Preven-
   tive and Social Medicine', 27, 70-1.
4 McMullen, S. (1972), The Significance of the Early Stages of
   Illness as a Focus for Social Work Help, 'British Journal of
   Social Work', 2/3, 255-67.
5 Ferguson, R.S. (1970), Roles of Medicine and Social Science in
   Future Health Service of Britain, 'British Journal of Medical
   Education', 4/2, 158-63.
6 Silver, G.A. (1963), 'Family Medical Care', Harvard University
   Press, Massachusetts.
7 McKay, A. et al. (1973), Consumers and a Social Services
   Department, 'Social Work Today', 4/16, 487-91.
8 'Social Work (Scotland) Act' (1968), HMSO, Edinburgh.
9 Department of Social Administration, Edinburgh (1969), 'Social
   Work in Scotland', University of Edinburgh.
10 Mayer, J.E. and Timms, N. (1970), 'The Client Speaks', Routledge
   & Kegan Paul, London.
11 Berger, P.L. (1967), 'Invitation to Sociology', Penguin, London.
12 Wootton, B. (1959), 'Social Science and Social Pathology', Allen
   & Unwin, London.
13 Plowman, D.E.G. (1969), What are the Outcomes of Casework?,
   'Social Work', 26/1, 10-19.
14 Timms, N. (1971), Research in Social Work, 'British Journal of
   Social Work', 1/3, 345-51.
15 Cooper, B. (1971), Social Work in General Practice: the Derby
   Scheme, 'Lancet', 1/7698, 539-42.
16 Holson, C.J. and Crayburn Davis, W. (1970), Social Work in a
   Group Medical Practice, 'Psychosomatics', 11/4, 355-7.
17 Ghan, L. and Road, D. (1970), Social Work in a Mixed Group
   Medical Practice, 'Canadian Journal of Public Health', 61/6,
   488-96.

18 Crown, S. (1972), Psychiatry and the General Medical Service,
    'Medicine', 10, 661-71.
19 Owen, J.H. (1972), The Social Worker Joins the Team, 'Australian
    Family Physician', 1/7, 393-6.
20 Olsen, R. (1974), From the Medical Journals, 'Social Work Today',
    5/13, 385-6.
21 Muras, H.J. et al. (1971), Who will Employ the Medical Social
    Workers?, 'Social Work Today', 1/10, 14-17.
22 Jefferys, M. (1965), 'An Anatomy of Social Welfare Services',
    Michael Joseph, London.
23 Linden, V. (1972), To What Extent is Information about Social
    Servises Available to People in Social Need?, 'T. Norske
    Laegeforen', 92/23, 1460-2.
24 The Royal College of General Practitioners (1972), 'The Future
    General Practitioner: Learning and Teaching', British Medical
    Journal, London.
25 Journal of the Royal College of General Practitioners (1973),
    'The Health Team', Report 16, 42-9.
26 Scobbie, J.S. (1972), Better Patient Care in an Organised
    Practice, 'Health Bulletin', 30/3, 201-3.
27 Warin, J.F. (1968), Health Centres in Oxford, 'Medical Officer',
    119, 115-9.
28 McGregor, A. (1969), Total Attachment of Community Nurses to
    General Practices, 'British Medical Journal', 3/5665, 291-3.
29 Rowland, A.J. et al. (1970), Evaluation of Home Nurse Attach-
    ment in Bristol, 'British Medical Journal', 4/5734, 545-7.
30 MacGregor, S.W. (1971), 'The Evaluation of a District Nursing
    Attachment in a North Edinburgh Practice', Scottish Health
    Service Studies No.18, Edinburgh.
31 Richardson, I.M. (1974), General Practitioners and District
    Nurses, 'British Journal of Preventive and Social Medicine',
    28, 187.
32 Carstairs, V. (1966), 'Home Nursing in Scotland', Scottish
    Health Service Studies No.2, Edinburgh.

Chapter 7

FACTORS ASSOCIATED WITH SYMPTOMS AND REFERRAL

'When you can measure what you are speaking of and express it in numbers, you know that on which you are discoursing. But when you cannot measure it and express it in numbers, your knowledge is of a very meagre and unsatisfactory kind.'   Lord Kelvin (1824-1907)

This chapter describes the associations found on simple correlation between the dependent variables for symptom prevalence and referral behaviour, and the independent variables. The statistical procedures are outlined in the introductory section, before discussing in the following three sections the findings for each of the dependent variables as they appear across the top of Appendix IV, which summarizes the results. The final section of the chapter reviews the correlation results from the point of view of the various factors taken into account by the independent variables.

INTRODUCTION

The relationship between the dependent variables shown in Figure 1.4 and each of the independent variables listed in Figure 1.5 was analysed using breakdown and cross-tabulation programmes.(1)   The ten dependent variables for symptom prevalence and referral behaviour (Figure 1.4), were first broken down as continuous variables to give their mean values for the categories of each independent variable and the F statistic was used to test the significance of the difference between the means.(2,3) The symptom frequencies and referral scores were then tabulated in a grouped form with the independent variables, and the chi-squared test was used to assess the significance of the cross-tabulations.(1,4)

   The results of these procedures are summarized in Appendix IV which shows those correlations which were significant at the 0.05 level as measured by the two significance tests indicated above. The strength of the associations in terms of significance values or correlation coefficients have not been included, because such measures depend upon the degrees of freedom involved and the level of measurement. Not only did variables have different numbers of

categories, but several of the independent variables were purely
nominal scales in which even rank order correlation coefficients
would have had little meaning. It must also be emphasized that
significant correlations as measured by the F statistic and chi-
squared test do not necessarily imply causation, but simply that
there is a probability that the two variables concerned are associated in some way. The nature of that association is another matter,
and therefore positive results pose questions rather than provide
answers.

The numbers of significant correlations are given at the margins
of Appendix IV, both for dependent and independent variables, and
show considerable differences. These were at least partly due to
the different numbers involved. For instance, the frequency of
physical symptoms was applicable to all 1,344 subjects, whereas the
referral scores for social symptoms only involved a minority of
adults with social symptoms for which the referral was known. While
it is not very helpful to compare the number of significant correlations for the measures of symptom prevalence and referral behaviour,
it is interesting to look at the frequencies of such correlations
for each independent variable. This gives some idea of the comparative importance of factors which might be associated with symptom
prevalence and referral behaviour.

It is not surprising that numbers of present illnesses, medicine
taking, and length of interview should have correlated with symptom
frequencies and referral behaviour, but that factors such as the
age of the house and family planning did not. What is more interesting was the obvious importance of employment status (particularly
unemployment), whereas factors such as social class and basic
amenities appear to have had much less relevance. Measures of
personality, mobility, and smoking also correlated with most of the
dependent variables, whereas intelligence, time of year, and which
practice people belonged to, seem to have had little bearing on
numbers of symptoms or referral behaviour.

Out of almost two thousand separate correlation procedures, 500
(27 per cent) were significant at the 0.05 level. It would not be
feasible to reproduce the figures for all of these, but the results
are reviewed below, first for the symptom frequencies and referral
scores, and then as a summary of the main groups of independent
variables with examples from some of the main factors which emerged.

CORRELATIONS WITH SYMPTOM FREQUENCIES

Almost two-thirds of the independent variables gave a significant
result on either breakdown or cross-tabulation with the number of
physical symptoms per person. Many of these associations were
either due to variables measuring the same thing, such as the number
of present illnesses, or to factors which were likely to be the
result of physical symptoms, such as the use of medical services and
medicine taking. In either case significant correlations could not
be considered as causal. The frequency of physical symptoms broadly
increased with age and was higher for females than males, though not
significantly so. As shown by Figure 7.1, women in the 30-44 age-
group had the largest number of physical symptoms, and children had

by far the least. Other significant sociographic variables indicated that people who were separated or divorced, unemployed due to
illness, had left school at an early age, or whose religious
allegiance was passive, were more likely to have an increased
number of physical symptoms.

Owner-occupiers and those living in more recent housing had fewer
physical symptoms, and those living at high densities, or on their
own, had significantly more. Cigarette smoking, and a high neuroticism score were also associated with an increased number of physical
symptoms. The relationship between mobility and the presence of
physical symptoms was complex, but in general those who had made
frequent moves, or who came from outside Glasgow especially from
Ireland, appeared to have significantly more physical symptoms.
The number of physical symptoms increased directly with other
measures of ill health, including the frequency of other symptoms,
and also with the use of both medical and social work services.
There was no clear relationship between symptom gradings and the
number of physical symptoms, but those with high frequencies tended
to be assessed as having poor social adjustment and high incongruous
referral scores.

The frequency of mental symptoms was significantly higher for
women than for men, with the middle-aged being the main age-groups
affected, as shown by Figure 7.2. Unemployment, especially due to
illness, and the lack of any active religious allegiance, were
associated with significantly more mental symptoms, as was living in
the fifth floor or above of high rise flats compared to other types
of housing. There was no clear relationship with other measures of
housing or mobility. Those who were separated or divorced tended
to have more mental symptoms, and there was a consistent social
class gradient from social class I to V, with the latter having the
most mental symptoms, but neither of these associations was significant. As with physical symptoms, the number of mental symptoms
increased with other measures of ill health, with the use of
medical and social work services, and with a poor assessment for
social adjustment. It is interesting that those who had difficulty
in contacting their doctor, or who had criticisms of the health
centre or the interview, or whose previous experience of doctors
and hospitals was ranked as bad - all had significantly higher
frequencies for mental symptoms. Not surprisingly, high neuroticism
scores and low extroversion scores were significantly related to an
increased number of mental symptoms. A high frequency of mental
symptoms was also associated with adults who tended not to seek
medical advice and who made incongruous referrals, especially those
who were part of the medical symptom 'iceberg'.

Several studies have suggested that psychiatric illness tends to
increase in women and with age,(5,6) although some kinds of mental
illness may be commoner in the younger age-groups,(7,8) and in this
survey it was the middle-aged rather than the elderly who had most
mental symptoms. Unemployment and low socio-economic status have
been related to mental illness in Ireland (9) and America,(10) but
these findings probably reflect the different coping capacities of
individuals rather than any intrinsic relationship to social class.
(11) Although those born and brought up in Ireland tended to have
more mental symptoms in the present survey, as in a study from

London,(12) these differences were not significant and there was little to indicate any overall increase in mental symptoms as has been reported from other studies, for instance of immigrant minorities.(13,14,15)

Comparatively few independent variables gave significant correlations with the frequency of behavioural symptoms in children. This was partly because of the smaller numbers involved, partly because several variables did not relate to children, and partly because the symptoms themselves were less well defined. Questions relating to personality, intelligence, and perception of services were asked of respondents answering for children rather than of the children themselves. The age distribution of behavioural symptoms is shown in Table 3.1. There were more behavioural symptoms amongst boys, as has been reported from studies of psychiatric illness.(16) The number also increased for those living in high rise flats, and in tenements with outside toilets, but these trends were not significant. The frequency of behavioural symptoms did increase significantly with the number of present illnesses or disabilities, and with the frequency of physical symptoms. Other studies have also reported an association between emotional disorders and physical illness in children.(17) Respondents who were not parents, who knew how to contact a social work department, who had been sterilized or who had personal problems, especially relating to the law or alcohol, all reported significantly more behavioural symptoms in children. The tendency for behavioural problems in children to be referred for informal advice was reflected in such symptoms being associated with low formal referral scores, and being part of the symptom 'iceberg'. Lay referral was also reflected in the significant association between behavioural symptoms and an increase in unprescribed medicine taking, as well as with respondents who were aware of sources of neighbourhood advice.

Social symptoms were most prevalent amongst the 30-44-year-olds and also amongst women, as shown by Figure 7.3, although sex was not a significant variable. Perhaps the elderly were less likely to have difficulties with children and teenagers, although other studies have emphasized the extent of psycho-social problems in old age.(18, 19) Factors which indicated a lack of personal stabilities such as unemployment, separation or divorce, neuroticism, absence of religious allegiance or contact with relatives, and several moves - all correlated significantly with the frequency of social symptoms. Measures of the physical environment, such as living at high densities and lack of basic amenities, were also associated with significantly more social symptoms. All the variables for symptom frequencies and social referral increased with the number of social symptoms, as did other estimates of poor health and the use of health and social services.

CORRELATIONS WITH THE TENDENCY TO REFER FORMALLY

The tendency to refer medical symptoms for professional advice was most marked in the young and the old as shown by Figure 7.4. The age-group differences were significant, unlike the sex differences, in which females scored more than males. A similar preponderance

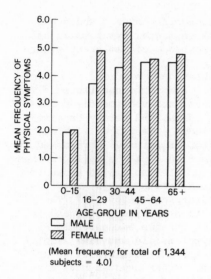

FIGURE 7.1 Age-sex distribution
of physical symptoms

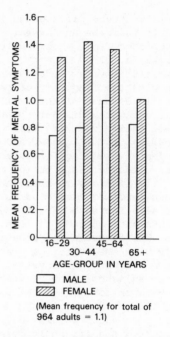

FIGURE 7.2 Age-sex distribution
of mental symptoms

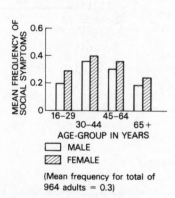

FIGURE 7.3 Age-sex distribution
of social symptoms

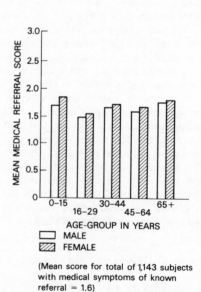

FIGURE 7.4 Age-sex distribution
of tendency to refer medical
symptoms formally

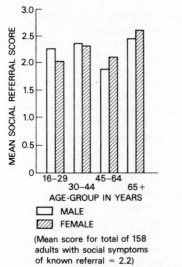

FIGURE 7.5   Age-sex distribution of tendency to refer social symptoms formally

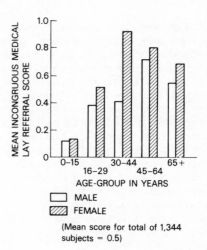

FIGURE 7.6   Age-sex distribution of medical symptom 'iceberg'

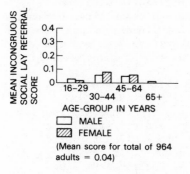

FIGURE 7.7   Age-sex distribution of social symptom 'iceberg'

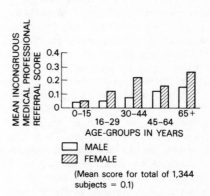

FIGURE 7.8   Age-sex distribution of medical symptom 'trivia'

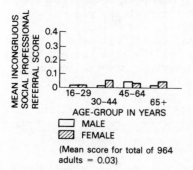

FIGURE 7.9   Age-sex distribution of social symptom 'trivia'

of children, the elderly, and women has been reported from surveys
of the work load in general practice,(20,21) and studies of
referral patterns to doctors in several different countries have
confirmed that women consult more often than men.(22,23,24,25)
Medical referral was considerably higher in unemployment due to
illness, but reduced if unemployment was not due to illness. There
was no significant trend or correlation with social class, although
increased medical referral has been associated with a lower social
class in England,(21) and the reverse in America (26,27) where the
use of medical services is more likely to be related to income.(28)
There were no significant correlations with measures of housing,
although those living on the upper floors of high flats tended to
have higher mean medical referral scores. Mobility did, however,
seem to be related to medical referral, which was significantly
higher for frequent movers, for those who had recently registered
with their doctor, and those whose previous residence had been overseas.

Medical referral increased with other estimates of ill health
and the use of medical and social services, and was also significantly higher for both past and present cigarette smokers. But
access to the health centre in terms of time and method of travel
did not appear to affect the tendency to refer medical symptoms
formally, nor did measures of personality or intelligence. The
mean medical referral scores increased significantly with the
symptom grading scales, especially for pain and disability, but the
relationship with symptom frequencies was not linear. Those with
few or many physical symptoms were least likely to seek medical
advice, and in particular those with several mental symptoms had
low mean medical referral scores.

There were few significant correlations with the mean social
referral score, partly because only a minority of adults had social
symptoms. As shown by Figure 7.5, the mean score tended to increase
with age and for women, but the differences were not significant.
However, those in rented accommodation and those without inside
toilets were significantly more likely to refer their social symptoms
formally. A study of social work clients in England,(29) also
reported a preponderance of the elderly, women, and tenants,
especially with bad housing conditions. These problems may be
related to the use of other services in view of the significant
correlations in the present survey between high mean social referral
scores and increased numbers of home visits by doctors, prescribed
medicine taking, and contacts with other helping agencies. The
mean social referral score correlated significantly with the
frequencies of mental and social symptoms, but the relationship was
not linear in that those with few or many symptoms had the lowest
scores. As for medical referral, this suggests that those with
multiple psycho-social problems tended to remain part of the
'iceberg'. For both medical and social referral the associations
between the mean scores and the incongruous scores were as expected,
in that those who were part of the 'iceberg' did not seek professional advice whereas those with 'trivia' did.

CORRELATIONS WITH THE 'ICEBERG' AND 'TRIVIA'

Females were more likely than males to be part of the medical symptom
'iceberg', especially the middle-aged, followed by the elderly, as
shown by Figure 7.6. Perhaps mothers with growing families felt
less able to seek professional advice for their symptoms, and
several studies have drawn attention to the extent to which disease
may not be reported with increasing age. This may be partly due
to fear,(30) and partly because such conditions, though treatable,
may be considered an inevitable part of growing old.(31) Those who
were unemployed, who had no higher education or active religious
allegiance, and those in social classes III and IV, were significantly more likely to be part of the medical symptom 'iceberg'.
Conversely, owner-occupiers and those living in larger dwellings
had significantly lower incongruous medical lay referral scores.
Studies from America (32,33) also support the impression from the
present survey that low socio-economic status is associated with a
tendency not to seek medical care. The significant correlations
with housing and mobility suggest that it was those from Glasgow
in the worst tenanted accommodation, and with frequent moves within
the city, who were most likely to be part of the medical symptom
'iceberg'. As these were also the characteristics of the non-
responders, it is probable that the survey results underestimated
the extent of this 'iceberg'. In contrast, those from overseas had
the lowest incongruous medical lay referral scores. It is interesting that it was the more neurotic and less intelligent who did not
trouble their doctors when perhaps they should have done, rather
than the other way round.

A long walk to the health centre, preference for the doctor's
previous surgery, and lack of a telephone, all seemed to discourage
medical referral. The incongruous medical lay referral scores
increased with the number of past and present illnesses, and also
with the numbers of both prescribed and unprescribed medicines being
taken. The tendency to be part of the medical symptom 'iceberg'
increased with the prevalence of symptoms, but was inversely
proportional to the other two medical referral scores. However,
about 7 per cent of those in the medical 'iceberg' also referred
medical 'trivia'. This suggests that for some there is no simple
pattern of behaviour to account for non-utilization of medical
care, and that even for one person different types of referral may
co-exist depending on the symptoms involved.

The age-sex distribution of the social symptom 'iceberg' is
shown in Figure 7.7, which indicates that, unlike the medical symptom
'iceberg', the elderly were the least likely to be involved, and in
fact there were no women over 65. There were comparatively few
significant correlations, partly because of the smaller numbers.
Those who were unemployed had significantly higher incongruous
social lay referral scores, as did the more neurotic and those who
smoked cigarettes. There were no clear associations with measures
of mobility and housing conditions.

Those in the social symptom 'iceberg' were more likely to be part
of the medical symptom 'iceberg' as well, and to have significantly
more mental and social symptoms. The situation was complex, however,
because there were significant correlations between the social

symptom 'iceberg' and a tendency to have been to a social worker or
to know someone else who had done so. Although the time span for
these latter variables was a year, whereas for social symptoms it
was only the past two weeks, it seems probable that there were
different referral patterns for different problems. For instance,
financial difficulties were the commonest social symptom found on
the survey, whereas those who were part of the social symptom
'iceberg' tended to have seen social workers about children.

The tendency to refer 'trivia' for medical advice increased with
age and for women, as shown in Figure 7.8. It was also significantly higher for the retired, separated or divorced, unemployed, or
those who had left school early. A preponderance of the divorced
and widowed amongst those making excessive demands was reported in
one study of general practice,(34) but other studies have found no
personal or social differences between patients considered in need
of treatment and those who were not.(35) There was a social class
gradient, with those in social class V being the most likely to
refer 'trivia', but the differences were not significant. Incongruous medical professional referral scores were lowest amongst
owner-occupiers, and significantly higher for those living in one
room or in households of one or two people only. The scores for
those living on the top floors of high rise flats were three times
those on the lower four floors, and the differences were almost
significant at the O.O5 level. The tendency to refer medical
'trivia' increased directly with the number of moves, and was lowest
for those who came from Glasgow or from overseas.

Incongruous medical professional referral scores increased with
estimates of past and present ill health, and also with other
measures of the use of health services. The significant correlations with personality and smoking habits were not linear and
suggested a complex relationship, as did the associations with
doctor preference and access to the health centre. The tendency to
refer medical 'trivia' formally increased directly with the
frequency of physical, mental, and also social symptoms. This
supports the impression that social symptoms tended to be referred
for professional advice, though not necessarily to social workers.
These results also underline the fact that there are often latent
reasons for the apparently unnecessary referral of trivial medical
symptoms. A survey of general practice in Holland (36) concluded
that the great majority of adults had some other reason for seeking
medical advice than the presenting complaint. Another study of
people labelled as 'problem patients' by their doctors found that
such patients considered themselves to be more ill, and had more
interpersonal and social difficulties.(37) In the present survey,
those who referred 'trivia' for medical advice tended to think that
their present health was bad and that they had a number of illnesses
and disabilities.

Those who referred social symptom 'trivia' tended to be female
and middle-aged as indicated by Figure 7.9, but there were few
significant correlations. The incongruous social professional
referral score was significantly higher for those who were unemployed
due to illness, and also for those who lived on the fifth floor or
above of high flats. High scorers tended to be introverted, to
rate their present health as poor, and to be taking several

prescribed medicines. They were also significantly more likely to
be disgruntled with their experiences of medical care and the health
centre. Those who referred social symptom 'trivia' for formal
advice tended not to know what social workers did and to have been
to other helping agencies. They also had significantly more
physical and social symptoms. Unlike the incongruous referral
scores for medical symptoms, the two scores for social symptoms
were mutually exclusive, and no one who was part of the social
symptom 'iceberg' also formally referred social symptom 'trivia'.

SUMMARY OF CORRELATIONS

The correlation results are now discussed by looking at the findings
for the independent variables which appear down the margins of
Appendix IV, as headings for each of the rows.

Introductory variables

The differences in symptom frequencies and referral scores between
the eight practices from which the subjects were drawn, were not
significant, although some of the variations were considerable,
especially for the tendency to refer medical 'trivia'. Nor did
a significant seasonal pattern emerge for any of the dependent
variables. The importance of employment status was probably partly
due to the fact that the coding for this question also took into
account age (e.g. child, student, retired) and sex (e.g. housewife).
However it was those who were unemployed, especially if due to
illness, who stood out for both symptoms and referral behaviour.
Figure 7.10 shows that unemployment due to illness was associated
with the highest frequencies for physical, mental and social symptoms.
This group also had the highest scores for the tendency to refer
medical symptoms formally on the one hand, and for the medical
symptom 'iceberg' on the other. This suggests two different
attitudes towards ill health by the unemployed, with perhaps some
more anxious to return to work than others. Age was the next most
important sociographic variable, especially when combined with sex
to give age-sex groups as shown by Figures 7.1 to 7.9. Females
tended to have higher scores than males, except for children's
behavioural symptoms, but the differences were only significant for
mental symptoms and for the referral of medical 'trivia'. Marital
status, like employment status, had a strong element of age, but
nevertheless those who were separated or divorced had the highest
symptom frequencies and were the most likely to refer medical
'trivia' as indicated by Figure 7.11. Education was also age
related, with those who left school early tending to have higher
scores. Those whose religious allegiance was only passive of what-
ever denomination, had consistently higher symptom frequencies as
shown by Figure 7.12, and were more likely to be part of the medical
symptom 'iceberg', than those with an active religious allegiance.
There were no clear social class gradients apart from a tendency for
mental symptoms to increase towards social class V, and for a significant excess of social class III and IV in the medical symptom
'iceberg'.

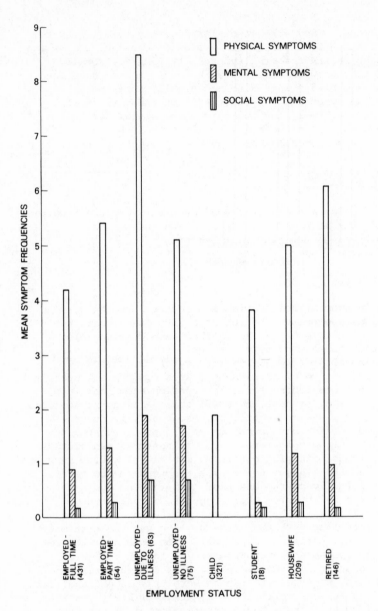

FIGURE 7.10   Employment status and symptom frequencies

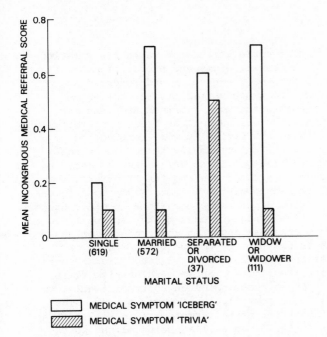

FIGURE 7.11 Marital status and the medical symptom 'iceberg' and 'trivia'

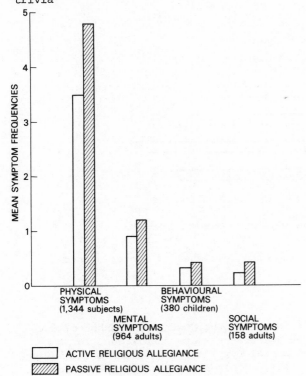

FIGURE 7.12 Religious allegiance and symptom prevalence

Housing

The most frequent significant correlations for variables relating
to housing were those for number of rooms and number of people in
a household. In general, symptom frequencies and referral scores
were inversely proportional to these variables, so that those
living in one room or alone had the most symptoms and were more
likely to seek professional advice, as well as being over-represented
in the 'iceberg'. When these two variables were combined to give
density of people per room, the relationships tended to be non-
linear in that both low and high densities had higher scores; the
one reflecting single people on their own and the other crowded
families. Owner-occupiers had consistently lower symptom frequencies and referral scores than others, whereas those in older houses
or who lacked basic amenities tended to have higher scores. However there were no strong associations with the presence or absence
of basic amenities such as own toilet, hot water, and bath or
shower. In contrast all the dependent variables had higher scores
for those living in the fifth floor or above of high-rise flats
when compared to other types of housing, such as traditional four-
storey tenements or the lower four floors of tower blocks. The
differences were significant for mental symptoms (Figure 7.13), and
also for social symptom 'trivia', as well as being almost so for
medical 'trivia'.

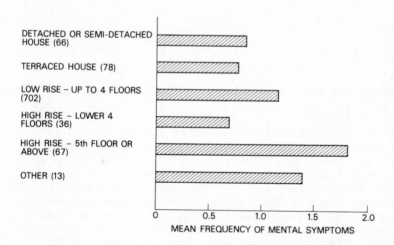

FIGURE 7.13 Type of housing and prevalence of mental symptoms

Mobility

Most of the dependent variables increased with the number of moves
made by a subject, and the differences were significant for the
frequency of physical and social symptoms, and also for the medical
referral scores (Figure 7.14). The relationship of the dependent
variables to length of residence and length of registration was less

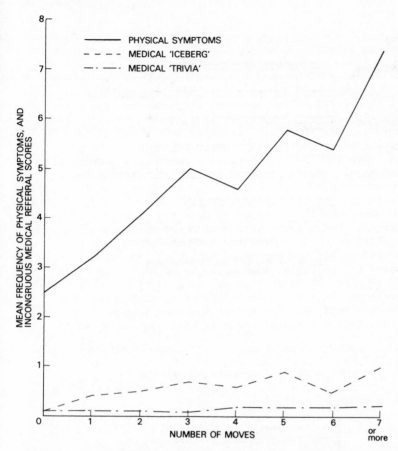

FIGURE 7.14 Mobility, symptom prevalence, and medical referral
(1,344 subjects)

clear, because both factors were influenced by age and mobility.
Those who had recently moved or registered with their doctor were
significantly more likely to seek medical advice. A long period of
registration with a family doctor was compatible with frequent
moves within the Glasgow area, and it is interesting that the prevalence of physical symptoms was highest for those whose previous
residence was in Glasgow, as well as for frequent movers and those
who had been registered a long time with their doctor. The prevalence of physical and mental symptoms was highest for subjects who
were born or brought up in Ireland, (Figure 7.15). Those whose
previous address had been in Ireland had twice the number of mental
symptoms compared with others. Although the tendency to seek medical advice was most marked in those from overseas, mainly from the
Indian sub-continent, this group did not have higher frequencies of
physical or mental symptoms. Contact with relatives did not seem
to be an important factor, apart from an increased number of social
symptoms amongst those who saw little of their relatives.

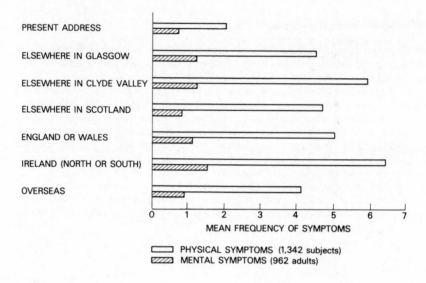

FIGURE 7.15   Place of birth and symptom prevalence

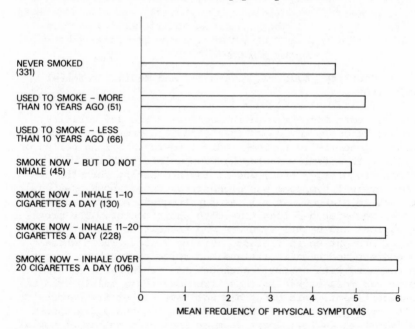

FIGURE 7.16   Cigarette smoking and prevalence of physical symptoms

Past and present health

In general both symptom frequencies and referral scores increased
with estimates of present and past ill health such as the number of
stays in hospital. The variables relating to smoking assessed the
number of cigarettes smoked, as well as whether subjects inhaled,
and whether they had given up smoking and if so when. The frequency
of physical symptoms increased significantly with the amount smoked
(Figure 7.16) and for those who inhaled. Significant correlations
with medical referral scores indicated that those who used to smoke,
but had given it up, and present-day heavy smokers were the most
likely to seek medical advice, whereas those who were currently
smoking a moderate amount were the least likely to refer medical
symptoms formally. Perhaps the tendency to seek medical advice
reflected health consciousness on the one hand, and a result of ill
health on the other.

Personality and intelligence

The personality and intelligence scores were derived from short
tests completed by most respondents including those answering for
children. The age and relationship of those interviewed about
children were also recorded, but the only significant correlation
was the tendency for more behavioural symptoms to be reported by
those who were not parents. The neuroticism score increased with
all the adult symptom frequencies (Figure 7.17), and also for those
in the medical symptom 'iceberg', who in addition had lower intelligence scores than others. Conversely, those who referred medical

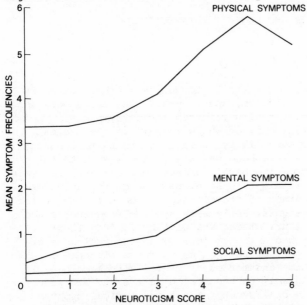

(1,238 subjects for physical symptoms, and 888 adults for mental
and social symptoms)

FIGURE 7.17   Neuroticism and symptom prevalence

'trivia' appeared to be less neurotic, and it was an unexpected
finding that a tendency to seek medical advice was not associated
with a neurotic personality but rather the other way round (Figure
7.18).   Subjects with low extroversion scores had significantly
more mental and social symptoms.   Introverts also tended to have
higher incongruous referral scores, especially for social symptom
'trivia'.   There were no significant correlations for the short
test of medical knowledge, and in general estimates of intelligence
seemed to be much less likely to be associated with symptom
frequencies or referral behaviour than was personality.

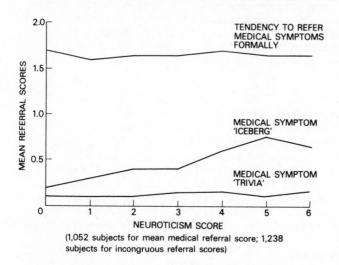

(1,052 subjects for mean medical referral score; 1,238
subjects for incongruous referral scores)

FIGURE 7.18   Neuroticism and medical referral

Use of medical services

The number of surgery and home visits tended to increase directly
with all the dependent variables, and in particular there were more
home visits to those who formally referred social symptoms.   Those
with several physical symptoms, or who were part of the medical
symptom 'iceberg', were more likely to rely on others to contact
their doctor.   Lack of a telephone was associated with both the
medical and social symptom 'iceberg', whereas medical 'trivia' were
referred more by those with a telephone; but the differences were
not significant.   The method of travel used in reaching the health
centre only correlated significantly with symptom frequencies and
not with referral behaviour.   Those who went by car had fewer
symptoms, but those who had a longer journey to the health centre
were more likely to be part of the medical symptom 'iceberg'.   When
the two variables for time and method of travel were combined, it
was those who had a long walk to the health centre who had significantly more mental or social symptoms; and the medical symptom
'iceberg' was also associated with a long walk or bus journey to
the health centre as indicated by Figure 7.19.

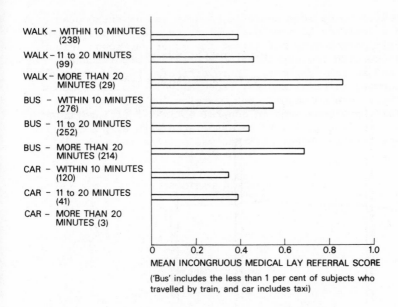

WALK – WITHIN 10 MINUTES (238)
WALK – 11 to 20 MINUTES (99)
WALK – MORE THAN 20 MINUTES (29)
BUS – WITHIN 10 MINUTES (276)
BUS – 11 to 20 MINUTES (252)
BUS – MORE THAN 20 MINUTES (214)
CAR – WITHIN 10 MINUTES (120)
CAR – 11 to 20 MINUTES (41)
CAR – MORE THAN 20 MINUTES (3)

0   0.2   0.4   0.6   0.8   1.0
MEAN INCONGRUOUS MEDICAL LAY REFERRAL SCORE

('Bus' includes the less than 1 per cent of subjects who
travelled by train, and car includes taxi)

FIGURE 7.19   Travel to health centre and the medical symptom
              'iceberg'

Perception of medical services

Those whose previous experience of doctors and hospitals was graded
as bad tended to have higher scores for the dependent variables,
especially for the frequency of mental or social symptoms, and they
were also more likely to refer medical symptom 'trivia' as shown by
Figure 7.20. This latter correlation was the opposite to what
might have been expected, and suggests that the perception of medical services was the result rather than the cause of referral
behaviour. The same applied to difficulties in contacting a doctor,
which were mentioned more often by those who tended to refer
symptoms formally as well as by those with higher symptom frequencies.
There was, however, a significant correlation between the medical
symptom 'iceberg' and a preference for one's doctor's previous
surgery over the health centre. Those who had criticisms of the
health centre also had significantly more mental and social symptoms.
Two attitude questions about the use of home remedies and action if
in doubt about a symptom produced no clear associations, but a
preference for one's own doctor did correlate significantly with a
tendency to refer medical symptoms formally.

Medicine taking

In general, the taking of prescribed medicines increased with both
symptom frequencies and referral scores, including the medical

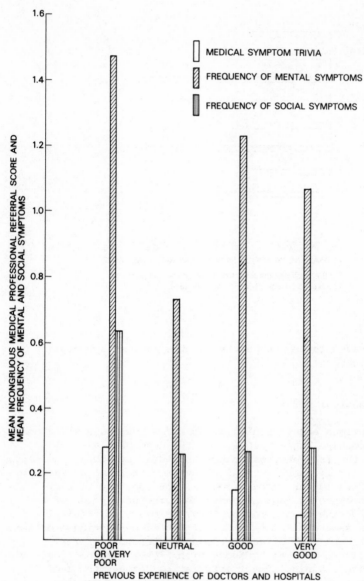

FIGURE 7.20   Previous experience of medical care, 'trivia' and
symptom prevalence

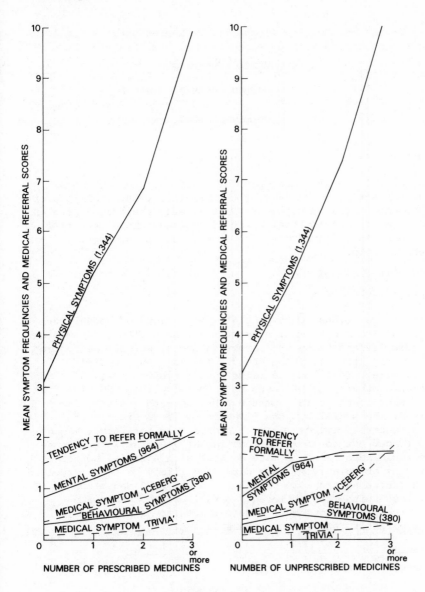

FIGURE 7.21 Medicine taking, medical symptoms and referral

symptom 'iceberg' as shown in Figure 7.21. Repeat prescriptions
tended to be associated with more behavioural symptoms and the
formal referral of social symptoms. Unprescribed-medicine taking,
also tended to increase for subjects with higher symptom frequencies
and referral scores, especially among those who were part of the
medical symptom 'iceberg', but not for behavioural symptoms, as
indicated by Figure 7.21.

Use of social worker

The values of all the dependent variables were greater for those
who had seen a social worker during the previous year. Domestic or
coping problems amongst adults were particularly associated with an
increased frequency of physical symptoms, whereas those reporting
mental and behavioural symptoms were more likely to see social
workers about children.

Perception of social work

The answers to questions about people's perceptions of social work
showed a significant correlation between a tendency to refer medical
symptoms formally and those who perceived social workers as dealing
with the elderly, whereas those who did not know what social
workers did were more likely to refer social symptom 'trivia'. Subjects who knew others who had been to a social worker had significantly more mental and social symptoms, but were themselves likely
to be part of the social symptom 'iceberg'. Those with several
physical or mental symptoms, or with high scores for formal medical
referral, tended not to know the location of a social work department, and would have tried to make contact with a social worker by
asking friends or relatives; they were also likely to have perceived
the health centre as the main point of contact with social work. In
contrast, those with more children's behavioural symptoms and
especially social symptoms were likely to contact a social work
department directly, and to know where it was.

Other sources of assistance

The use of helping agencies apart from doctors and social workers
increased with all the dependent variables except for the frequency
of children's behavioural symptoms. There were significantly
higher frequencies of physical and social symptoms amongst those
who used other agencies for problems involving the elderly or
housing, whereas illness was the main reason given by those in the
medical symptom 'iceberg', and difficulties with children by those
in the social symptom 'iceberg'. Subjects with more behavioural
and social symptoms were the most likely to mention informal individuals as sources of neighbourhood advice. Those with mental
symptoms tended not to know anyone to whom they could turn for
advice, and people in the medical symptom 'iceberg' were most
likely to mention themselves as sources of neighbourhood help.

Family planning

The questions on family planning were incidental to the main objectives of the survey, but nevertheless reflected an important aspect
of community health. Those who had been sterilized were more likely
to have high symptom frequencies, especially for children's behavioural and social symptoms. A tendency to refer medical symptoms
formally also correlated significantly with those who had been
sterilized or who were on the pill. Subjects with several social
symptoms were significantly more likely to obtain contraceptive
supplies from their own general practitioners. Those who were part
of the medical symptom 'iceberg' tended to use no contraception and
not to go anywhere for advice or supplies. People with higher
frequencies of mental or social symptoms were more likely to be
dissatisfied with family planning facilities.

Interviewer assessments

All four of the subjective assessments for home conditions, social
adjustment, cooperation and reliability tended to be rated as poor
by the interviewers, for subjects with higher symptom frequencies
and referral scores. An interesting exception was that those who
referred medical symptom 'trivia' were significantly more likely to
be rated as 'good' for the condition of the home and social adjustment; and they were also considered to be more uncooperative.

The interview

The length of the interview increased with the values of all the
dependent variables. There were more favourable comments on the
interview from those who were part of the symptom 'iceberg', and
also from those with fewer medical symptoms. Unfavourable comments
were associated with a tendency to refer symptoms formally, and
also with an absence of physical symptoms. The presence of others
during the interview correlated significantly with the frequency of
physical symptoms and medical referral scores. Those interviewed
alone, or with a spouse present, had more physical symptoms than
when parents or children were present; these differences were at
least partly due to age. In general, the presence of husbands or
wives was associated with a decreased tendency to seek medical
attention, in contrast to the presence of siblings or children.
Those who said at the end of the interview that they had other
personal matters troubling them had significantly more physical,
mental and children's behavioural symptoms.

Symptom grading scales

The mean grading scales for pain, disability and perceived seriousness were all directly proportional to the tendency to refer medical
symptoms formally, but the only significant correlation with symptom
frequencies was an inverse relationship between the mean pain score

and the number of mental symptoms. As pain was defined in terms of worry for mental symptoms, presumably the more mental symptoms a person has the less he says he worries about each one. A similar relationship was found between mental symptoms and the amount of worry or inconvenience caused by social symptoms. Although there were several significant correlations with the mean duration score, the relationships with symptom frequencies were complex and no clear pattern emerged. This was partly because the duration score measured both periodicity and length of time. In general, the longer the mean duration of medical symptoms, the less likely subjects were to seek medical advice, although the tendency to be part of the medical symptom 'iceberg' also decreased with long-standing symptoms.

Symptom frequencies and referral scores

On the whole symptom frequencies and referral scores tended to rise together, which might be expected in view of the inter-relationship of different types of symptoms and the fact that more symptoms will lead to more referrals whether incongruous or not. One exception was that the incongruous lay referral scores were inversely proportional to other referral scores because of the way the symptom 'icebergs' were defined. The other exception was a non-linear relationship between mean referral scores and symptom frequencies. Those with few or many symptoms were the least likely to seek professional advice, perhaps because multiple symptoms tended to make individual symptoms seem less severe.

The large number of correlations reviewed above reflect the extent of the data and the complexity of factors involved in symptom prevalence and referral behaviour. The breakdown and cross-tabulation procedures are simply ways of describing in more detail the available information in a quantitative form that indicates the amount of association between variables. The probability that these associations may be due to chance is assessed by statistical tests of significance. Significant correlations, however, do not imply causation, but rather suggest lines of enquiry that might be worth pursuing. It is also possible to gain some idea of the relative importance of different factors by multivariate analysis, as described in the next chapter. But whether for simple correlations or multivariate techniques, results have to be interpreted in the light of the data and its limitations. There are considerable difficulties in quantifying aspects of human behaviour and the environment in which we live, but without an attempt being made our knowledge would remain 'of a very meagre and unsatisfactory kind'.

REFERENCES

1 Nie, N.H. et al. (1970), 'Statistical Package for the Social Sciences', McGraw-Hill, USA.
2 Scientific and Social Sciences Program Library (1973), 'SPSS Update Manual, 1973 Revision', Edinburgh University.
3 Blalock, M.M. (1972), 'Social Statistics', McGraw-Hill, Kogakusha, Tokyo.

4   Documenta Geigy (1970), 'Scientific Tables', J.R. Geigy,
    Switzerland.
5   Bentz, W.K. and Edgerton, J.W. (1972), Demographic Correlates
    of Psychiatric Illness, 'Research Previews', 19/1, 7-13.
6   Schwab, J.J. et al. (1973), Depressive Symptoms and Age,
    'Psychosomatics', 14/3, 135-41.
7   Plutchik, R. (1973), Psychiatric Symptoms, 'Journal of American
    Gerontological Society', 21, 519.
8   Hare, E.H. et al. (1971), The Age Distribution of Schizophrenia
    and Neurosis, 'British Journal of Psychiatry', 119, 445-58.
9   Walsh, D. (1969), Social Class and Mental Illness in Dublin,
    'British Journal of Psychiatry', 115, 1151-61.
10 Warheit, G.J. et al. (1973), An Analysis of Social Class and
    Racial Differences in Depressive Symptomatology: A Community
    Study, 'Journal of Health and Social Behaviour', 14, 291-9.
11 Mechanic, D. (1972), Social Class and Schizophrenia, 'Social
    Forces', 50/3, 305-9.
12 Kelleher, M.J. et al. (1974), Assessment of Neurotic Symptoms
    in Irish Female Patients, 'British Journal of Psychiatry', 124,
    554-5.
13 Bagley, C. (1971), Mental Illness in Immigrant Minorities in
    London, 'Journal of Biosocial Science', 3/4, 449-59.
14 Bagley, C. (1971), The Social Aetiology of Schizophrenia in
    Immigrant Groups, 'International Journal of Social Psychiatry',
    17/4, 292-304.
15 Haberman, P.W. (1970), Ethnic Differences in Psychiatric
    Symptoms Reported in Community Surveys, 'Public Health Reports',
    85, 495-502.
16 Wing, J.K. et al. (1968), 'Camberwell Psychiatric Case Register
    - third report', MRC Social Psychiatry Research Unit, London.
17 Mumford, E. (1972), Physical, Social and Emotional Problems in
    an Elementary School, 'Paper at 3rd International Conference of
    Social Science and Medicine - Elsinore'.
18 Blank, M.L. (1971), Recent Research Findings on Practice with
    Ageing, 'Social Casework', 52/56, 382-9.
19 Kennie, A.T. et al. (1973), The Quality of Life in Glasgow's
    East End, 'Age and Ageing', 2, 46-54.
20 Oliemans, A.P. and De Waard, F. (1969), Morbidity in General
    Practice, 'Huisarts Wetensch', 12/9, 309-15.
21 Marsh, G.N. and McNay, R.A. (1974), Factors Affecting Workload
    in General Practice, 'British Medical Journal', 1/5903, 319-21.
22 Anderson, R. et al. (1968), Perceptions and Response to
    Symptoms of Illness in Sweden and the US, 'Medical Care', 6/1,
    18-30.
23 Namey, C. and Wilson, R.W. (1972), Age Patterns in Medical Care,
    Illness, and Disability, USA, 1968-69, 'Vital Health Statistics',
    10/70.
24 Holst, E. and Scocozza, L. (1973), Socio-Medical Survey of
    Doctor-Patient Contacts, 'Social Science and Medicine', 7/9,
    729-43.
25 Office of Population Censuses and Surveys (1973), 'The General
    Household Survey', HMSO, London.
26 Koos, E.L. (1954), 'The Health of Regionville', Columbia
    University Press, New York.

27 Elder, R. and Ascheson, R.M. (1970), Social Class and Behaviour
    in Response to Symptoms of Osteo-arthritis, 'Millbank Memorial
    Fund Quarterly', 48, 449-502.
28 Bice, T.W. et al. (1972), Socio-Economic Indicators and Use of
    Physician Services, 'Medical Care', 10/3, 261-71.
29 McKay, A. et al. (1973), Consumers and a Social Services
    Department, 'Social Work Today', 4/16, 487-91.
30 Johnson, M.L. (1972), Self-Perception of Need amongst the
    Elderly: an Analysis of Illness, 'Sociology Review', 20, 521-31.
31 Working Party on Elderly People at Risk (1974), 'Final Report',
    Age Concern, Edinburgh.
32 Ludwig, E.G. and Gibson, G. (1969), Self-Perception of Sickness
    and the Seeking of Medical Care, 'Journal of Health and Social
    Behaviour', 10/2, 125-33.
33 Hyman, M.D. (1970), Some Links between Economic Status and
    Untreated Illness, 'Social Science and Medicine', 4, 387-99.
34 Jacob, A. (1969), The Social Background of the Artificial
    Practice, 'Journal of the Royal College of General Practitioners',
    17/78, 12-16.
35 Thomas, K.B. (1974), Temporarily Dependent Patients in General
    Practice, 'British Medical Journal', 1/5908, 625-6.
36 Brouwer, W. and Touw, O.F. (1974), Analysis of the Pre-Medical
    Period, 'Huisarts Wetensch', 17/1, 3-15.
37 Fabrega, H. et al. (1969), Low Income Problem Patients,
    'Journal of Health and Social Behaviour', 10, 334-43.

Chapter 8

MULTIVARIATE ANALYSIS

'The assumptions introduced to explain a thing must not be
multiplied beyond necessity.'   William of Occam (1280-1349)

This chapter presents the findings from the multivariate analysis,
first of all indicating the methods used, and then discussing the
results for the symptom frequencies and referral scores, of which
the details are given in Appendix V.   The approach is essentially
descriptive and does not presuppose hypotheses, which would be
implicit in partial correlation procedures of which there could
potentially be an enormous number.   The results are reviewed in
the final section in the context of a conceptual framework for the
findings.   The quantitative results of the regression equations are
therefore used in two ways.   First, the regression coefficients
indicate the relative importance of individual independent variables,
and second, the changes in variance produced suggest the extent to
which the prevalence of symptoms and referral behaviour are affected
by various factors.

INTRODUCTION

The results of bivariate analysis as presented in the preceding
chapter are difficult to interpret in view of the complexity of the
data and the number of factors involved.   Significant correlations
might be due to intervening variables, which on the other hand
might mask genuine causal relationships.   In addition, such correlation procedures give little idea of the relative importance of
independent variables, especially when interacting with each other
in relation to a dependent variable.

   In order to gain some perspective on the information available,
the relationship between the independent variables and each dependent variable was analysed by SPSS computer programs for multiple
regression.[1]   Such techniques require assumptions to be made
which often stretch the quality of survey data, but do make it
possible to study the effects of a number of different factors at
the same time.   One such general assumption is that the relationship

between variables is linear; this may not be so and therefore a significant correlation might disappear in a regression equation unless special techniques are used. For instance, on cross-tabulation there was a significant relationship between an increased frequency of physical symptoms and those living at both high and low densities, with moderate densities being associated with the fewest symptoms. Such a non-linear relationship would have little effect on a linear regression equation, irrespective of the strength of the bivariate correlation.

Another important assumption is that there are equal intervals between the categories of ranking scales, so that these can be regarded as interval scales. It is not feasible to treat nominal scales as if they were interval scales, but it is possible to create dummy variables for those categories of nominal variables which seemed to be important from the correlations.(2) The following nine dummy variables were created for regression analysis: separated or divorced; unemployed not due to illness; owner-occupier; living in the fifth floor or above of high-rise flats; walking to the health centre; contacting the doctor by telephone; knowing someone else who had been to a social worker; knowing how to con-tact a social worker; knowing the location of a social work depart-ment.

The absence of significant correlations on bivariate analysis did not necessarily exclude variables from multivariate analysis, because associations may have been masked by intervening factors. However variables which were peripheral to the main aims of the survey, such as family planning, were not included in the regression analysis, nor were factors which did not seem to be important or for which there were alternative measures. In general, only vari-ables which might be causal to the dependent variable concerned were included in the regression equations. These causal factors could be grouped under the following broad headings: biological; physical environment; social environment; mobility; stress; past medical history; present health; perception of services.

Biological factors were innate personal characteriseics such as age and sex, and also measures of personality and intelligence. The physical environment included variables related to housing, and also cigarette smoking for the prevalence of symptoms in adults. The social environment was represented by social class, religious allegiance, and contact with relatives. Mobility was assessed by number of moves, place of origin, previous residence, and length of time at present address.

Unemployment and separation or divorce were included as stress factors for adults, while for children the personality and relation-ship of those answering for them were used instead. The intellig-ence scores of respondents for children were considered as part of the social environment for behavioural symptoms rather than as stress factors. Past medical history was represented by the number of previous illnesses and stays in hospital.

The remaining two groups of factors for present health and per-ception of services were only used in the regression equations for referral behaviour because such variables either assessed the same thing as symptom prevalence or were a result rather than a cause of symptoms. Present health was measured by a self-estimate of health

and number of present illnesses, together with the grading scales
for medical and social symptoms respectively. For medical referral,
the perception of services was represented by variables for access
to and preference for doctors and the health centre. For social
referral, knowledge about access to social work and of others who
had been to social workers was used for the perception of services.

Measures of symptom prevalence and referral behaviour were not
used as independent variables in the regression equations because
many of the possible causal factors were strongly associated with
both symptoms and referral. In addition, the referral scores were
partly defined by the number of symptoms. When the symptom preval-
ences were included in the analysis for referral behaviour, these
accounted for a high proportion of the variability to the exclusion
of other factors which would otherwise have been strongly associated with referral, and therefore other estimates of present
health were included instead of symptom prevalence. The symptom
grading scales were only used in analysing the two scores for the
tendency to refer symptoms formally, but not for the incongruous
referral scores because these latter were defined in terms of the
grading of symptoms.

The computer programme for multiple regression proceeded in a
stepwise fashion by recursively constructing prediction equations,
one independent variable at a time.(1) At each step the variable
was entered that would have the highest predictive value in conjunc-
tion with the other variables already in the equation. Cases with
missing values were excluded from the analysis for that particular
variable. At the end of each multiple regression the programme
printed out a summary table with the independent variables shown in
the order in which they had been included in the equation. The
tables also gave the regression coefficients for the last step of
the equation together with the changes in variance produced as each
variable was added in turn. Whereas the change in variance produced at each step remained constant for each independent variable,
the regression coefficients could alter every time another variable
was added because of interaction between variables. The regression
coefficients shown therefore related to the final equation and
reflected the interactions of all the variables added. The programme
included default options, which meant that variables that made
little difference to the regression equation were excluded. The
default values were set very low because variables that made little
difference to the overall variance might still have affected other
variables in the equation by interaction.

The results of the final regression equations for each dependent
variable are given in Appendix V with an explanatory note. In the
sections below, the multiple regression analysis for each dependent
variable is described in turn, emphasizing those factors that had
significant regression coefficients, and indicating where these
differed from the simple correlations, thus reflecting the strength
of interaction effects.

REGRESSION FOR SYMPTOM FREQUENCIES

In the regression analysis for the frequency of physical symptoms,
22 variables were used of which 1 (social class) did not reach the
default values for inclusion in the regression equation. Of the
remaining 21 variables, the following 10 had significant regression
coefficients:
   Neuroticism score
   Number of short hospital stays
   Age
   Number of moves
   Number of cigarettes smoked
   Religion (passive allegiance)
   Sex (female)
   Birth and upbringing (away from Glasgow)
   Intelligence score (low)
   House ownership (tenant)
All of these variables had significant simple correlations with
physical symptom prevalence, except for the female sex and low
intelligence scores, which were more prominent on regression analysis. Those who had had a previous residence away from Glasgow, or
who had been in their present residence a long time, had significantly more physical symptoms on simple correlation, but these
relationships were reversed on regression analysis, probably because
of the age factor. The results suggest that personal characteristics such as age, sex, personality, and intelligence were important
factors in the prevalence of physical symptoms. Whereas cigarette
smoking might be causal, other variables such as hospital stays were
more associations. Mobility was also important and may reflect a
lack of personal stabilities like the absence of an active religious
allegiance. Tenants may also be less stable in terms of mobility
in Glasgow than owner-occupiers.

   In the regression analysis for the frequency of mental symptoms
in adults, 22 variables were used of which 2 (number of moves
and cigarette smoking) did not reach the default values for inclu-
sion in the regression equation. Of the remaining 20 variables,
the following 10 had significant regression coefficients:
   Neuroticism score
   Number of short hospital stays
   Sex (female)
   Age of housing (older)
   Unemployment - not due to illness
   Age
   Intelligence score (low)
   Religion (passive allegiance)
   Social class (lower)
   High rise flats (living in)
Of these variables, age, intelligence score, age of housing and
social class were not significant on simple correlation. As for
physical symptoms, personal characteristics were also significant
factors in the prevalence of mental symptoms, but cigarette smoking
and mobility were not. Instead, measures of housing such as older
housing or high-rise flats seemed more important, as were variables
relating to the social environment like social class, unemployment,
and lack of religious allegiance.

The housing variables were not the usual measures of bad
housing, such as overcrowding and lack of basic amenities, but
factors suggesting the social rather than physical environment.
The high-rise flats were all comparatively recent and therefore
the variable for older houses represented a different aspect of
housing. However, those who were rehoused in new flats were likely
to have come from older housing and therefore the two variables
were complementary in that they both referred to a similar population of people in the lower occupational groups. Both types of
housing might lead to anomie and anxiety; in high-rise flats
because of the lack of social contact in unfamiliar surroundings,
and in older houses because of the dereliction caused by planning
blight in slum clearance areas. Perhaps when the physical amenities
of the home are adequate, the less perceptive are more likely to
express the social strains of such situations as mental symptoms.
Many writers have emphasized the psychosocial aspects of disease,
(3) and in particular the importance of life events for the prevalence of mental symptoms.(4,5) Surveys in America suggest that
mental illness is more associated with stress factors in adult life
rather than childhood,(6) and depressive disorders have been related
to social environments which block opportunities and aspirations.(7)
It is not easy, however, to distinguish cause from consequence when
studying the social correlates of mental illness. The present
analysis provided descriptive pointers rather than causal answers,
which would require longitudinal studies to identify social factors
that preceded mental illness.(8)

There were 20 variables used in the regression analysis for the
frequency of behavioural symptoms in children, of which 7 (age of
housing, previous residence, number of moves, contact with relatives,
number of previous illnesses, age of respondent, and basic amenities) did not reach the default values for inclusion in the regression equation. Of the remaining 13 variables, the following 3 had
significant regression coefficients:
   Number of long hospital stays
   Relationship of respondent (not a parent)
   Neuroticism score of respondent
Neither the number of long hospital stays, nor the neuroticism
score of the respondent gave significant correlations on bivariate
analysis, but a respondent who was not a parent was significant on
simple correlation. A stay in hospital of six months or more would
either be due to serious illness or birth injury. Physical illness
in children has been associated with emotional disturbance,(9) and
minimal brain damage may lead to behavioural disorders.(10) Long
hospital stays would also result in maternal deprivation, which has
been linked with disordered behaviour.(11) Such deprivation is
also suggested by the absence of a parent answering for the child,
and a high neuroticism scores for those answering would indicate
the possibility of unstable relationships. All these factors would
tend to lessen the security of children and increase the likelihood
of behavioural problems.

Again, 22 variables were used in the regression analysis for
the frequency of social symptoms in adults, of which 3 (previous
residence, number of long hospital stays, and house ownership) did
not reach the default values for inclusion in the regression

equation. Of the remaining 19 variables the following 8 had signif-
icant regression coefficients:
   Neuroticism score
   Unemployment - not due to illness
   Age
   Separation or divorce
   Number of short hospital stays
   High rise flats (not living in)
   Religion (passive allegiance)
   Years in present residence (few)
Neither the absence of living in high-rise flats nor a short time
in the present residence was significant on simple correlation.
The factors that emerged as important correlates of social
symptoms on regression analysis seemed to relate to personal
instabilities in employment, in marriage, in a recent move, or in
lack of religious allegiance. Although not included in this
regression analysis there was a strong correlation between social
symptoms and the prevalence of mental symptoms which has been noted
in other studies.(12,13,14) Apart from increased density, factors
relating to bad housing conditions did not seem to be very important, although other surveys in Glasgow (15,16,17,18) and elsewhere
in the United Kingdom (19) have shown how measures of social
dysfunction cluster in areas of poor housing.

REGRESSION FOR THE TENDENCY TO REFER FORMALLY

As many as 32 variables were used in the regression analysis for
the tendency to refer medical symptoms formally. Of these only 2
(number of short hospital stays, and time to health centre) did
not reach the default values for inclusion in the regression
equation. Of the remaining 30 variables the following 12 had sig-
nificant regression coefficients:
   Number of present illnesses
   Mean seriousness score
   Age (younger)
   Mean pain score
   Self-estimate of present health (poor)
   Mean disability score
   Birth and upbringing (away from Glasgow)
   Difficulty in contacting doctor
   Neuroticism score (low)
   High rise flats (living in)
   Unemployment - due to illness
   Doctor preference (own doctor or partner)
Of these, age, birth and upbringing, neuroticism and living in
high-rise flats did not have significant correlations on bivariate
analysis. In addition the sign of the coefficients changed
between simple correlation and regression analysis, for age and
number of previous illnesses. The relationship with age alone was
not linear in that it was the young and the old who were the most
likely to refer medical symptoms formally (Figure 7.4), and an
overall inverse relationship to age emerged on regression analysis.
Apart from age the most important factors associated with the

formal referral of medical symptoms were concerned with the perception of symptoms and present health.

Surveys in America (20) and also cross-cultural studies (21)
have confirmed the present finding that perceived seriousness is a
major determinant of physician utilization and the use of health
services. Prior experience of a situation also lessens the likelihood of seeking medical attention by reducing anxiety and uncertainty.(22) After perceived seriousness, pain seemed a more important trigger than disability for seeking medical advice. In
general the perception of symptoms appeared to be a stronger determinant of referral than the perception of sources of assistance.
Certainly a preference for one's own doctor or partner was associated with a higher referral score, but the association with
difficulty in contacting a doctor would seem to be the result
rather than a cause of medical referral. The fact that neuroticism
and unemployment due to illness were both inversely proportional to
the tendency for medical referral, is perhaps contrary to some
preconceptions, but fits in with the finding of high neuroticism
scores amongst the medical symptom 'iceberg' rather than 'trivia'.
The associations with an origin outside Glasgow and living in high
flats are echoed in the findings for medical symptom 'trivia', and
raise intriguing questions about the role of anomie as a determinant of referral behaviour.

A total of 25 variables were used in the regression analysis
for the tendency to refer social symptoms formally. Of these, 5
(contacts with relatives, intelligence score, birth and upbringing,
separation or divorce, and knowledge about the nearest social work
department) did not reach the default values for inclusion in the
regression equation. Of the remaining 20 variables, the following
3 had significant regression coefficients:

   Neuroticism score (low)
   Number of previous illnesses
   Basic amenities (lack of)

None of these was significant on simple correlation. As for medical
referrals, it was the less neurotic who were more likely to refer
social symptoms for formal advice. The importance of ill-health and
bad housing in the referral of social symptoms was also emphasized
by these results. Although contact with other helping agencies was
not causal to social referral and therefore was not part of the
regression analysis, this variable did correlate strongly both on
simple and multivariate correlation, reflecting the diversity of
referral for social problems.

REGRESSION FOR THE 'ICEBERG' AND 'TRIVIA'

There were 28 variables used in the regression analysis for the
medical symptom 'iceberg'. Of these, 3 (years in present residence, number of present illnesses, and basic amenities) did not
reach the default values for inclusion in the regression equation.
Of the remaining 25 variables, the following 6 had significant
regression coefficients:

Neuroticism score
Number of previous illnesses
Self-estimate of present health (poor)
Age
Number of moves
Sex (female)

Of these only the variable for female sex was not significant on
simple correlation. While the medical symptom 'iceberg' correlated
significantly with the number of short hospital stays and a previous residence outside Glasgow on bivariate analysis, the direction of these associations changed on multivariate analysis and
ceased to be significant. Apart from estimates of poor past and
present ill-health, it was the more neurotic who were part of the
medical symptom 'iceberg', which was also associated with increasing
age, mobility, and females. Low intelligence scores and a long bus
journey to the health centre were also more likely for those in the
medical 'iceberg', but the regression coefficients for these factors
were not significant.

There were 24 variables used in the regression analysis for the
social symptom 'iceberg'. Of these, 3 (sex, religious allegiance,
and number of moves) did not reach the default values for inclusion
in the regression equation. Of the remaining 21 variables the
following 5 had significant regression coefficients:

Number of previous illnesses (few)
Neuroticism score
Unemployment - not due to illness
Age
Knowledge about others contacting social worker

Of these only the number of previous illnesses was not significant
on simple correlation. In addition the regression coefficients
indicated a direct association with increasing age, whereas cross-
tabulation indicated mainly the middle-aged with an overall negative correlation coefficient. As with the medical symptom
'iceberg', the social symptom 'iceberg' was associated with a high
neuroticism score. Unemployment and knowledge of others who had
been to a social worker were probably reflections of the social
environment rather than causal factors.

There were 28 variables used in the regression analysis for
medical symptom 'trivia'. Of these, 4 (contact with relatives,
preference for health centre, doctor preference, and walking to the
health centre) did not reach the default values for inclusion in
the regression equation. Of the remaining 24 variables the following 9 had significant regression coefficients:

Number of present illnesses
Separation or divorce
Age
Experience of doctors and hospitals (poor)
Years in present residence (few)
Difficulty in contacting doctor
Number of short hospital stays
Sex (female)
Number of long hospital stays (few)

Three of these were not significant on simple correlation, namely
recent moves, difficulty in contacting a doctor, and few long

hospital stays. In addition, the variables for self-estimate of
present health, previous residence, and neuroticism, were significant on simple correlation with coefficients of the opposite sign.
It is not surprising that those who referred medical symptom
'trivia' considered that they had a number of illnesses and that
they tended to be older and female. The associations with separation or divorce and a recent move, suggest that psycho-social
problems may have been the reason for referring medical 'trivia'.
The contrasting significance of short and long hospital stays is
hard to interpret. But the variables for difficulty in contacting
a doctor and poor experience of doctors and hospitals suggest the
result rather than causes of referral behaviour.

There were 24 variables used in the regression analysis for
social symptom 'trivia'. Of these, 3 (number of moves, present
illnesses, and knowledge about nearest social work department) did
not reach the default values for inclusion in the regression
equation. Of the remaining 21 variables, the following 3 had
significant regression coefficients:

High-rise flats (living in)
Number of present illnesses
Birth and upbringing (in Glasgow)

Only the variable for living in high flats was also significant on
simple correlation, and suggests that social 'trivia' were perhaps
a reaction to the anomie of tower blocks especially for those who
had been born and brought up in another part of Glasgow. As well
as considering that they had a number of present illnesses, those
referring social symptom 'trivia' also felt that they had a number
of present illnesses and tended to be unemployed though not due to
ill health.

REVIEW OF REGRESSIONS

Although a wide range of variables was used in the regression
equations, these accounted for less than a third of the variance
of any of the dependent variables, as indicated by Figure 8.1.
This is perhaps not surprising in view of the nature of the dependent variables all of which were synthesizing computations from
the initial data involving considerable simplification, so that,
for instance, differences between individual symptoms could not be
taken into account. In addition, the assumptions about interval
scales and linear relationships generally implicit in linear multivariate analysis tend to suppress correlations and if anything
flatten the data, typically leaving much of the data unexplained.
The highest proportion of variance was explained for the prevalence
of physical and mental symptoms which had the most precise methodologies. The social symptom 'iceberg' and 'trivia' had the least
amount of variance accounted for, partly because of the small
number of incongruous social referrals.

Very few of the independent variables seemed individually to
cause an appreciable amount of variation. The main value of the
regression analysis was, therefore, partly negative in that it
indicated those factors which were probably not important correlates of the dependent variables after allowing for a wide range of

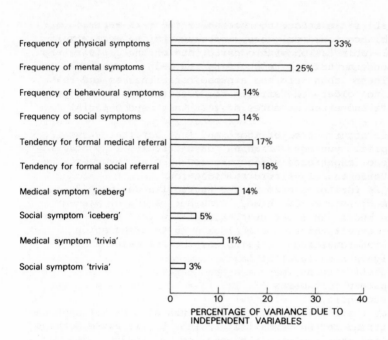

FIGURE 8.1   Change in variance due to independent variables

possible interaction effects. Some variables, such as unemployment,
seemed less important on multivariate as opposed to bivariate
analysis, whereas other variables, such as social class, assumed
a greater prominence when interacting with other factors.

The regression equations also highlighted variables which main-
tained significant coefficients on both simple correlation and
multiple regression. For instance, the neuroticism score emerged
as the foremost independent variable in half the regression equations, and was a significant factor in both symptom prevalence and
referral behaviour (except for the referral 'trivia'). The consis-
tency of these results strongly refutes the stereotype of neurotic
personalities bothering medical and social work services, with the
professional implication that much of such referral is unnecessary.

It was not surprising that age and sex remained significant
variables on regression analysis, nor that previous hospitalization
was strongly associated with symptom prevalence, and cigarette
smoking with physical symptoms. Less expected was the continued
prominence of measures of mobility, and also of living in high
flats and an absence of active religious allegiance. These variables were significant for symptom prevalence as well as for
referral behaviour, and raise questions about the place of instability as a cause of ill health.

Another way of gaining some perspective on the relative importance of the various factors involved is to look at the changes in
variance produced by the different groups of variables as described
in the introduction to this chapter. To a certain extent such
groupings are arbitrary, and the changes in variance depend partly
on the number of variables included in each group; although if

several variables are measuring the same thing then the relevant change in variance would only occur once and not be multiplied accordingly. Table 8.1 shows the percentage changes in variance for each dependent variable produced by the groups of independent variables. These groups provide a broad conceptual framework within which to compare the effects of different aspects of people and their environment on measures of ill health and referral behaviour.

Biological factors were the most important for the prevalence of mental and social symptoms. Personal characteristics also accounted for the largest amount of variance associated with the symptom 'iceberg'. Variables classified as biological were the second most important group for the prevalence of physical symptoms and also for the tendency to refer both medical and social symptoms formally. It seems, therefore, that personal characteristics are not only the major factors associated with the prevalence of symptoms but also with the likelihood of someone being part of the symptom 'iceberg'. The comparatively high level of mental symptom variance accounted for by biological factors, may have been partly due to questions in the personality test being similar to some of those used for psychiatric screening.

Measures of the physical environment achieved little prominence, except in relation to the formal referral of social symptoms. These variables, relating mainly to housing, appeared to make little impact on the prevalence of symptoms, with mental symptoms showing the most variation. The social environment seemed to have little effect on any of the dependent variables, with the prevalence of mental symptoms again being the most susceptible.

Mobility had most effect on the tendency to refer social symptoms formally and on medical symptom 'trivia', and perhaps surprisingly seemed more relevant to physical than to other types of symptoms. Measures of stress appeared to be mainly related to the prevalence of social symptoms in adults and behavioural symptoms in children, as well as to medical symptom 'trivia'. In many ways stress is an unsatisfactory concept when applied to factors impinging on people's lives, unless it is carefully defined. A better term might be social discontinuities as measured by such life events (23) as the loss of a job, separation or divorce, and number of moves. When viewed together in this way, variables relating to mobility and stress had most effect upon the prevalence of social symptoms and the referral of medical symptom 'trivia', with perhaps the former being a reason for the latter.

After biological factors, variables estimating past medical history accounted for the most overall variance. Previous ill health was the most important factor in the variability of physical and especially behavioural symptoms. The relationship of ill health to behavioural problems in children has already been noted. Previous ill health was also the most prominent factor in the tendency to refer social symptoms formally, and was again important in the medical and social symptom 'iceberg'. The relationship of past illness to social referral emphasizes the close connections that should exist between medical and social work services.

Measures of present health and the perception of services were only used in the multivariate analysis of referral behaviour

TABLE 8.1 Change in variance produced by groups of independent variables

| Groups of independent variables | Percentage change in variance | | | | | | | | | |
| | Symptom frequencies | | | | Tendency to refer formally | | 'Iceberg' | | 'Trivia' | |
	Physical	Mental	Behavioural	Social	Medical	Social	Medical	Social	Medical	Social
Biological	11.0	18.2	0.6	5.8	1.3	4.3	6.2	1.7	0.9	0.3
Physical environment	0.9	1.1	0.2	0.8	0.4	3.9	0.1	0.3	0.3	0.8
Social environment	0.9	1.0	0.5	0.9	0.1	0.4	0.1	0.2	0.1	0.2
Mobility	1.5	0.6	0.1	0.7	0.7	2.2	0.3	0.2	1.5	0.3
Stress	0.1	0.6	3.2	4.3	0.5	0.1	0.2	0.7	1.6	0.3
Past medical history	18.2	3.3	9.3	1.3	0.1	5.4	5.5	0.8	0.6	0.4
Present health	-	-	-	-	13.0	1.2	1.3	0.3	3.9	0.9
Perception of services	-	-	-	-	1.3	0.7	0.5	0.6	1.7	0.1

because present health assessed the same thing as symptom prevalence, for which the perception of services was hardly causal. As
might be expected, estimates of present health were the main factor
associated with the tendency to seek professional advice for medical
symptoms in general, as well as for medical 'trivia'. The perception of services did not emerge as an important aspect of referral
behaviour. The dependent variable most affected was the referral of
medical symptom 'trivia', but the nature of these correlations
suggested that the perception of services was often the result
rather than a cause of referral behaviour.

Multivariate analysis with a number of variables presents more
problems than answers. It has been used here mainly as a descriptive
device to show the interaction effects of possible causal factors,
and to indicate the extent to which the variability of symptom
prevalence and referral behaviour can be accounted for by the
available data. The picture that emerges is blurred and incomplete;
it reflects a lack not only of precision tools for data collection
and analysis, but also of adequate conceptual models. At the most,
multivariate techniques provide some pointers to the relevant
questions and hopefully help to distinguish the wood from the trees,
although not yet with the confidence of Occam's razor.

REFERENCES

1 Nie, N.H. et al. (1975), 'Statistical Package for the Social
   Sciences', 2nd Ed, McGraw-Hill, USA.
2 Moser, C.A. and Kalton, G. (1971), 'Survey Methods in Social
   Investigation', Heinemann Educational, London.
3 Lipowski, Z.J. (1969), Psychosocial Aspects of Disease, 'Annals
   of Internal Medicine', 71/6, 1197-206.
4 Myers, J.K. et al. (1972), Life Events and Mental Status: A
   Longitudinal Study, 'Journal of Health and Social Behaviour',
   13/4, 398-406.
5 Uhlenhut, E.H. and Paykel, E.S. (1973), Symptom Configuration
   and Life Events, 'Arch. Gen. Psych.', 28, 744-8.
6 Berkman, P.L. (1971), Life Stress and Psychological Well-being,
   'Journal of Health and Social Behaviour', 12/1, 35-45.
7 Linsky, A.S. (1969), Community Structure and Depressive
   Disorders, 'Social Problems', 17/1, 120-31.
8 Robins, L.N. (1969), Social Correlates of Psychiatric Illness:
   Can We Tell Cause from Consequence?, 'Res. Publ. Ass. Res.
   Nerv. Ment. Dis.', 47, 154-69.
9 Mumford, E. (1972), Physical, Social and Emotional Problems in
   an Elementary School, 'Paper at 3rd International Conference of
   Social Science and Medicine - Elsinore'.
10 Weiss, G. et al. (1971), Behaviour Symptoms and Young Children,
   'Arch. Gen. Psych.', 24, 409.
11 Bowlby, J. (1965), 'Child Care and the Growth of Love',
   Penguin, London.
12 Philip, A.E. and McCulloch (1966), Use of Social Indices in
   Psychiatric Epidemiology, 'British Journal of Preventive and
   Social Medicine', 20, 122-6.
13 Cooper, B. (1972), Clinical and Social Aspects of Chronic
   Neurosis, 'Practitioner', 208, 289-90.

14 Fitzgibbons, D.J. (1972), Social Class Differences in Patients'
    Self-Perceived Treatment Needs, 'Psychology Reports', 31, 987-97.
15 Ferguson, T. (1952), 'The Young Delinquent in His Social
    Setting', Oxford University Press, London.
16 Mansley, R.D. (1973), 'Housing and Social Deprivation',
    Planning Department, Corporation of Glasgow.
17 Rae, J.H. (1974), 'Family Circumstances and Location of the
    Socially Deprived', Planning Department, Corporation of
    Glasgow.
18 West Central Scotland Plan (1974), 'Social Issues - Supplementary
    Report 4', Glasgow.
19 Martin, I. (1971), Research into Social Problems in Liverpool,
    'Social Work Today', 1/11, 4-8.
20 Hulka, B.S. et al. (1972), Determinants of Physician Utiliza-
    tion, 'Medical Care', 10/4, 300-9.
21 Bice, T.W. and White, K.L. (1969), Factors Relating to the Use
    of Health Services: An Internal Comparative Study, 'Medical
    Care', 7/2, 124-33.
22 Banks, F.R. and Keller, M.D. (1971), Symptom Experience and
    Health Action, 'Medical Care', 9/6, 498-502.
23 Brown, G.W. (1974), 'Stressful Life Events: Their Nature and
    Effects', in Dohrenwend B.S. and Dohrenwend B.P. (eds), John
    Wiley, New York.

Chapter 9

IMPLICATIONS

'There is a need for more consumer research and citizen involvement
in National Health Service affairs.'   (Chief Medical Officer
                at the Scottish Home and Health Department, 1973)

'The personal social services are large scale experiments in ways of
helping those in need. It is both wasteful and irresponsible to set
experiments in motion and omit to record and analyse what happens.'
                                              (Seebohm Report, 1968)

The practical implications of the findings are discussed first in
relation to symptom prevalence and referral behaviour, and then from
the point of view of the provision of medical services and social
work. Next the theoretical implications are discussed, and finally
suggestions put forward for further research. The approach to
developing theoretical ideas is essentially inductive in that the
research results give rise to concepts, rather than using the data
deductively to prove or disprove particular hypotheses.

SYMPTOM PREVALENCE AND REFERRAL BEHAVIOUR

Many of the significant associations with measures of symptom prevalence and referral behaviour were as expected, but others were
not, especially some of the factors which emerged on multivariate
analysis. It is not surprising that previous hospitalization was
an important variable in the frequency of symptoms, but the prominence of the neuroticism score for all the dependent variables was
unexpected, not only in extent but also in direction.
    Personality is an abstract concept that implies an inherent
characteristic of individuals reflected in their reactions to the
world and those around them. A number of questionnaires have been
devised to measure personality, such as the one in the present
survey which, though short, has been extensively used and validated.
(1) The resulting scores, however, are only the replies to certain
subjective questions, and the relationship between the abstract concept and its measurement is too tenuous to allow causal inferences

to be drawn. The answers to the questions may have been determined
by the presence of symptoms rather than measuring a predisposing
factor. Of more practical interest was the strength and consis-
tency of the relationship between personality and referral behaviour,
which showed that it was the less neurotic who were more likely to
seek professional advice both in general and for 'trivia'. Conversely, it was the more neurotic who were most likely to be part of
the symptom 'iceberg'. In view of the size of this 'iceberg' for
medical symptoms when compared to the 'trivia', it seems that
official campaigns in the United Kingdom to encourage people 'not
to trouble their doctor unnecessarily' were misdirected. Perhaps
popular prejudices about the use of services tend to be defined by
professional expectations, which may not reflect population needs.

Age and sex were strongly associated with most of the dependent
variables, although perhaps less so on multivariate than on bivariate
analysis. Females had higher symptom frequencies, with the exception that boys had more behavioural symptoms than girls. Women were
also more likely to refer symptoms formally, as well as being over-
represented in the medical symptom 'iceberg'. In general, symptom
frequencies increased with age, as did incongruous referrals. Both
could be considered as failures of adaptation with advancing years.
Incongruous referrals might be partly due to lack of insight and
knowledge, but also an expression of attitudes developed over time.
It was the young who went more readily to doctors and the elderly
who were most likely to be part of the symptom 'iceberg', especially
for mental symptoms. The practical implications of this are that
changes in the provision of primary care should take into account
existing attitudes and patterns of referral. Improvements should
evolve from traditional points of contact rather than being radic-
ally new departures, and the reorganization of services should be
preceded by research into referral behaviour.

The correlation between the prevalence of physical symptoms and
cigarette smoking was not unexpected. The facts about smoking and
health have been alarmingly clear for some time.(2) Over 50,000
people a year die in the United Kingdom as a result of lung cancer,
heart disease, or bronchitis, caused or partly caused by cigaretts
smoking. This is about one-tenth of all deaths, and less than half
of these people have reached the age of 65. In Scotland a larger
proportion of the population smoke cigarettes and smoke more per
head than in the rest of Britain, and death rates are correspond-
ingly higher. Scotland has some of the highest known rates in the
world for lung cancer, which is a rare disease amongst non-smokers
even in industrial towns. One man in twelve dies from lung cancer
in Scotland, and in parts of Glasgow this proportion may rise to
one in eight;(3) with the encouragement of advertising, the rates
for women are also increasing. It is estimated that about three-
quarters of the mortality from chronic bronchitis, and one-quarter
of all deaths from ischaemic heart disease before the age of 65,
are due to smoking cigarettes.(2) The days lost through sickness
absence from bronchitis in Britain are about ten times those lost
from industrial disputes, and approximately 12 per cent of subjects
in the present survey had the symptoms of chronic bronchitis.
Ischaemic heart disease is the commonest cause of death in industrial societies, and again Scotland has a higher mortality than the

rest of the United Kingdom. In addition bladder cancer and peri-
natal mortality have been associated with cigaretts smoking. It
may not be feasible to alter people's age, sex, or personality, but
it is certainly possible to change smoking habits if only by differ-
ential taxation to encourage the far safer smoking of pipes and
cigars. Official failure to take effective action against the
smoking of cigarettes must rank as one of the most extraordinary
examples of self-deception and self-destruction in modern times.

A number of variables were used to assess mobility, and the
relationship between these measurements and the dependent variables
was complex. On regression analysis an increased number of moves
was associated with a higher frequency of physical symptoms and a
tendency to be part of the medical symptom 'iceberg'. A recent
move, on the other hand, correlated significantly with the prevalence of social symptoms and also a tendency to refer medical
'trivia', perhaps itself a reflection of social problems. Those
who were born and brought up away from Glasgow had more physical
symptoms and were more likely to seek formal medical advice, in
contrast to those originating from Glasgow who tended to refer
social symptom 'trivia'. A recent move or origins elsewhere might
result in temporary problems of adjustment, but frequent moves
suggest more chronic instability. Much of this mobility was within
the Glasgow area, which has a high proportion of local authority
tenants and where it has been estimated that one-quarter of the
population moves each year.(4) This mobility is largely due to
redevelopment, so that the resulting instability is a direct consequence of planning policies and a social situation where individuals have little choice over the fate of their homes. There may be
some grand overall design, but that is little consolation for those
left in the dereliction of planning blight or caught in the anonymity of rehousing. For all the tower flats and motorways, too much
of present-day Glasgow is a depressing indictment of the process of
urban planning. Some at least of this might have been avoided if
families and local communities had more control over, and responsibility for, their own environment.

Indeed, of all the housing variables, it was living in high-rise
flats above the usual four floors of Glasgow tenements that produced
the most significant regression coefficients, especially for the
prevalence of mental symptoms and the tendency to seek medical
advice. Mental symptoms were also associated with lower intelligence scores and social class, and it might be that those with less
insight tended to internalize the problems of a change to better
material conditions as mental symptoms. In contrast, social
symptoms and referral were associated with a lack of basic amenities
and with not living in new flats, perhaps because the more intelligent perceived social symptoms as arising from unfavourable
external circumstances. There are signs that tower blocks are not
being built to the same extent, if only because of expense, but it
might have been expected that they would create problems, especially
for families with young children. The results of this survey
suggest that such problems tend to become medically defined and
referred, although living in high-rise flats was also associated
with the small number of social symptom 'trivia'.

Unemployment not due to illness remained a significant variable

on regression analysis for the prevalence of mental and social
symptoms, as did separation and divorce for social symptoms and
the referral of medical 'trivia'. Both mental and social symptoms
appeared to be partly reactions to instabilities in a person's life,
such as the loss of a job or a spouse. Like mobility, these could
be thought of as social discontinuities or stressful life events.(5)
Lack of stability may also have been reflected in the prominence of
merely passive religious allegiance as a factor in the prevalence of
symptoms, which raises echoes of Durkheim's anomie.(6) The concept
of instability was particularly appropriate for children's behavioural symptoms. A long hospital stay and being looked after by
someone who was not a parent or with a high neuroticism score might
all affect a child's stability and produce behavioural problems.
Of these variables unemployment and mobility are the only ones
amenable to change by policy decisions. The two factors are not
unrelated, in that the forced mobility of rehousing may cause
unemployment,(7) while the inflexibility of public housing prevents
the voluntary movement of those seeking employment elsewhere.

It was not unexpected that variables relating to past and present
ill health were significantly associated with symptom prevalence and
referral behaviour, but it was perhaps surprising that the perception of services appeared to have comparatively little impact on
patterns of referral. Indeed most of the significant regression
coefficients for people's perceptions of services appeared to be the
result rather than a cause of their referral behaviour, for instance,
the difficulty in contacting doctors by those who tended to seek
medical advice or who referred medical symptom 'trivia'. Subjects
who preferred their own doctor or partner, however, were also more
likely to refer medical symptoms professionally. Although factors
relating to the perception of services were not prominent on
regression analysis, at a descriptive level the survey results had
implications for primary medical care and social work, which are
discussed below.

MEDICAL SERVICES AND SOCIAL WORK

The reorganization of the National Health Service in Britain, with
its emphasis on integrating primary and secondary care on a community basis together with preventive measures, implies that we know
where people are in the community. The inaccuracy of the health
centre records used for the present study raises considerable doubts
as to whether the quality of population data is sufficient for the
effective planning and delivery of community services. This is
particularly so in large conurbations, such as Glasgow, where there
is a high rate of internal mobility,(4) much of it due to housing
conditions.

There is no way of keeping track of this mobile population
without the legal means of recording changes of residence as in some
other countries, which would have political implications. Changes
of address within Glasgow can only be recorded if a patient attends
the health centre, because only births, deaths, and moves out of
the area are registered by the executive council. Even if information from both these sources was regularly used to update patient

record files, these would still be inaccurate because of the large
number of frequent movers within Glasgow who do not present for
medical care. In fact, the executive council lists for the health
centre practices contained several thousand fewer records than the
computer file. As the difference approximately accounted for those
who could no longer be effectively registered at the health centre,
there was probably no inflation of the official practice lists.

The computer file from which the survey sample was drawn contained the names, age, sex and address of patients registered with
the doctors practising from the health centre.(8)   Although com-
puters have been introduced in general practice for research (9)
and morbidity recording,(10) they are probably best used for small
amounts of information about large populations, rather than for
lengthy records for each individual case.(11)   Given the problem of
inaccuracies, the patient file in question might be usefully augmen-
ted by recording when patients were last seen, so that those who had
made no contact for some time could be followed up to find out if
they had moved or were part of the 'iceberg', which would be particularly relevant for at-risk groups such as the elderly.

On a larger scale it has been recommended that computerized data
banks should be set up in Scotland at area health board level with
central linkage and co-ordination for management purposes.(12)   Such
a system could make record linkage a reality, and have considerable
implications for preventive medicine, with effective follow-up and
at-risk registers linked to primary care from health centres. It is
unlikely that population data will ever be completely accurate, but
unless it is better than at present the objectives of a health
information system will not be properly realized. Although much can
be done by the routine checking of existing records and addresses,
this will not compensate for the deficiencies of present population
data, which raises wide issues concerning the use of identity numbers
and the registration of addresses. But unless the nettle is grasped,
health service information systems may turn out to be expensive
illusions built on shifting sands.

The findings of the present survey also have implications for the
spatial organization of health services.(13)   Some studies in Scotland suggest that it is more convenient and less costly for special-
ists to come to health centres rather than for patients to go to
hospital clinics,(14) and others have used estimates of population
location to decide the optimum position of urban health centres.(15)
It would seem better, however, to determine the siting of such health
centres from the basis of the present location of doctors' surgeries,
rather than on the presumed densities of a highly mobile population.
Amongst those interviewed, the average length of registration with a
doctor was twice as long as the average length of residence of seven
years, which was almost certainly an over-estimate due to bias from
the non-response rate. This means that the location of family
doctors is a much more stable point of reference than the location
of patients. Moreover, the information is accurate and easy to
acquire, which is more than can be said for the addresses of patients.

A rigid geographical definition of a health centre catchment area
also ignores two fundamental characteristics of the primary care
system in the United Kingdom. The first is that a family doctor has
continuing care for patients as they proceed through the family

life-cycle. This process involves mobility, but not necessarily a
change of general practitioner within a conurbation. The second
characteristic is the patient's choice of doctor, which may be
difficult in rural areas but not in cities or large towns. In fact,
the evidence suggests that patients exercise this choice to remain
with their family doctor even if they do change residence.

The survey data indicated that general practitioners were
preferred by the majority as the source of first contact, and that
their accessibility had not been impaired by practising from a
health centre. The main problems for patients related to their
access to a telephone and the appointments system. Although the
latter usually causes difficulties when first introduced,(16) there
did seem a case for reviewing arrangements. In particular, receptionists were placed in the position of being the first point of
contact and sometimes had to make decisions about priorities for
which they may not have had sufficient training or authority. At
times sickness certificates had to be backdated for a well person
who could not get an appointment when they felt ill, and sometimes
patients were placed in the position of having to request home
visits because of appointment delays. The availability of a doctor
to answer difficult incoming calls, and more flexibility in the
appointments system might have eased these problems.

The part played by social workers in dealing with the social
symptoms found in this survey appeared to be peripheral. Many
social problems were being formally referred in any case, and few
of them to social workers. There was also little awareness of how
to contact a social worker, and people were just as likely to go to
a health centre as to a social work department, although at the
time social workers were only attached to two of the eight practices. Such findings raise questions about the benefits of social
work to the community, in view of the costs of social work departments. The impetus for these developments seems to have come as
much from the need for social workers to professionalize social
work, as from the needs of the community. A similar comment could
be made about other professions, including medicine.

But there are also problems of methodology. Social symptoms
were defined in the present study as the subjective answers to four
open-ended questions about difficulties with children, difficulties
with other relatives, financial difficulties, and other difficulties
with day-to-day living. As definitions these are very hazy, and
what one person thinks is a social symptom may be quite different
from the views of another. While social workers may perceive
problems in terms of personal adjustments over time, clients may be
looking for practical help with immediate difficulties.(17)
Although the remit of social work departments is very broad, there
are many other formal sources for such practical help, as this
survey indicates. The difficulties of definition, however, do not
necessarily invalidate research or make it meaningless. Rather
they reflect the lack of clarity in service objectives and re-
emphasize the need for a critical and constructive evaluation of
social work.(18,19)

The desirability of cooperation between medical and social work
services is also underlined by the results of the present study.
Not only are social and medical problems inextricably interwoven,

but doctors, and the health centre in particular, were just as likely
to be perceived as sources of social referral as were social work
departments. Although reports from several different countries have
laid emphasis on the integration of medical care and social work,
(20,21,22,23,24,25,26) relationships between general practitioners
and social workers are sometimes marred by differences of approach
and role perception, as well as by problems of authority and confidentiality.(27) The idea that doctors should know more about social
and psychological problems has been recently stressed in medical
education (28) as well as by social workers,(29) although the concept
of medicine being concerned with the whole person is by no means
new. What is novel is the emergence of a new professional group,
and while the insights of behavioural science are important, the
main problem may be that doctors and social workers need to know
more about each other,(30) and the best way to achieve this is for
more integration in training.(31)

The situation might have been different had social case work
developed from general practice rather than forming a separate
service. If medical and social symptoms were viewed as a continuous spectrum of maladaptation, then the services concerned would
best be conceived as a coherent entity. This might throw a rather
different light on manpower planning than the present tendency to
equate the size and growth of distinct professional groups with the
quality and appropriateness of care.

Several health centres have opened in Scotland in recent years
(32) and their importance in an integrated health service has been
stressed.(33) Ideally general practitioners and other staff should
be involved at all stages in the design.(34) For instance, the
open-plan layout of reception areas has meant a lack of privacy for
both patients and receptionists who may need to talk in confidence.
(35) The size of health centres has sometimes been based on the
economics of facilities such as X-ray machines,(36) rather than on
the problems of access for patients and the implication of formal
management structures for large groups of family doctors. Although
the present study was not intended to be an evaluation of a health
centre, there is a need for this both before and after the introduction of new services.(37) For instance, the findings concerning
the appointments system illustrate the kind of feedback that has
implications for the provision of services, in this case the way in
which appointment delays may distort the demand for home visits and
the use of casualty services.

Users of public services often seem to be accepting and to think
in terms of the bother of complaining, rather than the duty of constructive criticism. Although many professional providers of
services are more open to suggestions than perhaps most recipients
realize, there is a gap in the institutional means of communication
which has not been effectively filled by the local health councils
in Scotland. Modern management does not always encourage constructive feedback, and the perceptions of planners and professionals
tend to be given precedence over the experiences of people. Perhaps
planning is too often seen as the production of static blueprints,
rather than the development of processes which can evolve and adapt.
The arguments for feedback do not rest on vague ideas about the
desirability of participation, but rather that without such

communication and the formal means of expressing it there is a lack
of flexibility and services are unable to adapt. The result is not
only frustration but inefficiency.

THEORETICAL IMPLICATIONS

The theoretical starting point of the present study was the concept
of the sick role,(38) and the importance of the social as well as
the medical response to illness.(39) Variations in sick role
behaviour have been associated with cultural differences,(40) illness frequency,(41) and family size.(42) Some have viewed illness
as a way of coping with failure,(43) and others have distinguished
between disease as a biologically altered state and illness that is
behavioural.(44) It has been suggested that the medical definition
of disease tends to limit the perception of people's troubles,(45)
and therefore illness behaviour should be converted to problem
behaviour as the main object of primary care.(46)
     Theoretical approaches to the utilization of services also imply
some perspective on the services themselves.(47) Differences
between the need and demand for services can reflect different
public and professional expectations.(48) These varying perspectives of patients and doctors might require new approaches from
professional training as part of an adaptive process.(49) There is
nothing immutable about the caring professions or the way in which
they practise. It has been pointed out that there is something
anomalous about social work splitting off from medicine at a time
when the problems of industrial living require an ecological perspective from services that have to locate themselves within the process
of social change.(50) This involves establishing priorities for
primary medical care (51) and the social services, within what has
been called social development planning.(52) Such plans should not
be stationary, but continual processes for which feedback from
patients and consumers is essential.(53) Without this the system
cannot adapt, with resulting imbalances between the availability of
services and need, which may become inversely proportional as
described by the inverse care law.(54)
     Illness behaviour can also be viewed as a form of adaptation.
Such a perspective seems more appropriate than considering illness
as a form of deviance,(55) which has been criticized on the grounds
that illness is, in fact, the norm rather than deviant.(56) The
findings of the present study suggest a complex interaction between
different types of symptoms, personal characteristics, and the
physical and social environment of which factors causing instability
were important. These included things like mobility, housing,
unemployment and marital breakdown, as well as specific behaviour
such as cigarette smoking. Symptoms can therefore best be looked at
in terms of people's adaptation to their environment, which implies
a broader view of aetiology than is usually defined within the
traditional research interests of the medical and social sciences.
Perhaps the boundaries between these disciplines should be less
important than they are. From the point of view of prevention, the
practical measures required lie largely outside the conventional
remit of medical and even social services, which function more by

picking up the pieces than by preventing the breakages from factors
like housing and unemployment.   These require political initiatives,
as was perceived in the last century by the pathologist Rudolph
Virchow who wrote that 'politics is medicine writ large'.

The idea that health is a form of biological and social adaptation is not new.(57)   It is an ecological concept relating health
and illness to the physical and social environment.   Moreover,
adaptation embraces not only disease but illness behaviour.   Adaptation also involves a time dimension, and implies that health and
illness are not just static but continual processes.(58)   The stage
at which health becomes illness depends not only on perspectives
and criteria, but also on the level of analysis.   This might be
biological and pathological, or behavioural.   The behavioural
aspects of health and illness are the adjustments that are an
essential part of adaptation.   These adjustments are mediated
through self-awareness and the perception of norms and sources of
assistance.

The results of regression analysis in the present survey suggest
that the perception of symptoms was more important than the perception of services in determining referral behaviour.   However, the
appropriateness of a particular symptom for referral was also
relevant, especially for the non-referral of mental symptoms.
Theoretically the concept of a functional 'sick role' as some kind
of consensus behaviour is an inadequate framework for the observed
facts.   One way of representing the marked variation in the extent
to which different types of symptoms were referred for formal advice
is shown in Figure 9.1.   The amount of formal referral is proportional to the distance from self.   Mental symptoms are closer to a
person's integrity than the physical symptoms of the body, and both
are more obviously part of an individual than social symptoms due
to external circumstances in society.   The extent to which people
internalize or externalize their perceptions of reality is similar
to the dichotomy between personal responsibility and the social

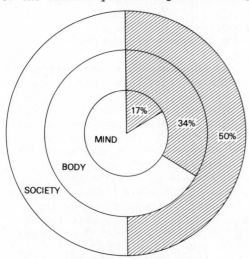

▨ FORMAL REFERRAL OF SYMPTOMS

FIGURE 9.1 Formal referral and distance from self

determinants of behaviour, between nature and nurture, and even between right- and left-wing views of society. In this model the place of contemporary medicine lies somewhere in the middle.

If symptoms can be viewed as an expression of maladaptation to the environment, then their referral may also show failure of adaptation, both on the part of individuals and society. Personal problems may not be perceived as being appropriate for professional advice. These perceptions may have been acquired in the past and failed to adjust to changing circumstances, or the services may simply not be available. Just as the adaptation of an individual depends on self-awareness, so the adaptation of society depends on social awareness. It is this social awareness, expressed through public concern, that enables society to adjust. Such adjustments tend to be slow and imperfect, partly because of the nature of political processes, and partly because of attitudes to change. Change means uncertainty, and in general people prefer the security of what they know, so that attitudes become out of step with reality as history changes behind our backs.

When it comes to the provision of services, further inertia may result from professional attitudes. These are formed in the past, handed on by the socialization of training, and continued in the interests of career patterns. The result may be a lack of fit between the services provided and the needs or demands of those being served.(59) This maladaptation is reflected by conflicting expectations as defined by the incongruous referral behaviour described in the present study, and depicted by Figure 9.2, in which professional definitions are assumed to correspond to the subjectivity severity of symptoms. Although the proportion of incongruous

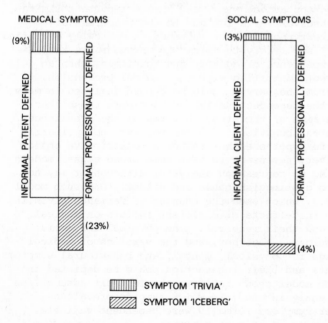

FIGURE 9.2 Lack of fit between services and recipients

referrals is greater for medical than social symptoms, there are
several sources of formal referral for the latter of which social
work is only one (Table 4.6). This can cause confusions over such
problems as homelessness, which in Scotland has been the responsibility of social work departments, who have found it necessary, for
instance, to pay expensive hotel accommodation for families evicted
by the housing department for rent arrears. Eventually these same
families have often been rehoused by the same department which made
them homeless in the first place.

FURTHER RESEARCH

The results of correlation and regression analysis have raised many
questions, some of which could be answered by further statistical
procedures, or by using other dependent variables. For instance,
individual symptoms or symptom clusters (60) could provide a basis
for analysis, and computer mapping could be extended to demonstrate
the geographical distribution of other variables. However, the
survey data was limited by its subjective nature, and by the fact
that there was no means of checking the information obtained,
although the questionnaire included some internal checks and
assessments of cooperation and reliability. Confidentiality pre-
cluded either return visits or the verification of answers against
other records. As well as posing problems of validity and repeat-
ability, a single interview makes it difficult to assess the time
dimension for the natural history of symptoms and the process of
referral.(58) In a sense, subjective answers about symptoms are
only valid for one person at one time, and a more important limita-
tion may have been observer variation due to the reactions of
respondents to different people. For instance, a medically qualified
interviewer was much less likely to elicit an unfavourable response
to questions about experience of doctors and hospitals, than an
interviewer who was not identified with the medical profession.
    The information from the survey could have been analysed in many
different ways, but the dependent variables used were those that
were relevant to the aims of the study in terms of the prevalence
of symptoms and referral behaviour. These aims were not primarily
formulated as discrete hypotheses but rather as descriptive objectives. It was, however, necessary to have some broad causal models
in view when embarking on regression analysis, although it may not
always be possible to distinguish cause and effect. One such model
is shown in Figure 9.3, which uses the changes in variance given in
Table 8.1 to compare the effects of different factors on medical
and social symptoms and their referral. The physical and social
environments are considered together, and the variance of medical
symptoms is an average for physical, mental, and behavioural symptoms.
The sequence of events and their interaction could be depicted in
several ways, but the model shown reflects the implicit assumptions
of the multivariate analysis used, in which symptom prevalence and
the tendency to refer symptoms formally were dependent variables
linked by other estimates of present health.
    The difficulties of interpreting the results of multiple
regression have already been discussed, but it is worth stressing

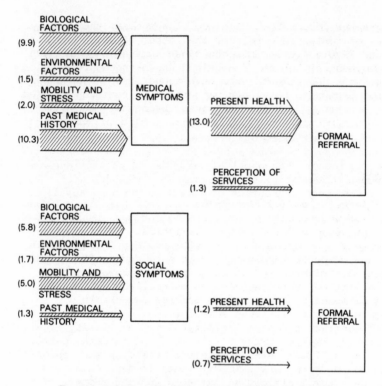

(The thickness of the horizontal lines is proportional to the change in variance, given in brackets, produced by the factors indicated)

FIGURE 9.3   Causal models of symptom prevalence and referral behaviour

again that significant associations are not necessarily causal. Both bivariate and multivariate analyses describe situations, whereas causal inference depends on interpretation, which might be made clearer by teasing out relationships with the plodding procedures of contingency table analysis.(61)   The present results suggest a number of specific hypotheses which could be tested in this way or made the objectives for further data collection.

There would seem to be a place for the kind of developmental research in primary care represented by the present study, which is not dominated by any one discipline.(62)   Although mainly descriptive, multivariate techniques introduce some perspective into a wealth of detailed information and significant correlations, which hopefully generate ideas for further research.   These ideas might vary from simple limited hypotheses to the middle-range theories of sociology,(63) like those suggested by the figures in this chapter. Projects could also be linked to specific management objectives and operational research.   This implies the possibility of intervention either in the provision of services or the prevention of causal factors in ill health.   Many of the causal factors which could be changed would require major policy decisions in areas such as housing, employment, and finance, which lie outside the scope of health and social services.   In particular, the environmental

reasons for individual maladaptation are nowhere more cruelly con-
centrated than in Glasgow;(64) and it is in tackling the causes
rather than the symptoms of malaise that the real priorities lie.

Ongoing evaluation of services should, however, be the concern of
the professions involved. This implies defining population needs,
(65) and providing information feedback both to and from the people
being served, as a continual process and an essential part of
management.(53,66,67) Such feedback might have implications, for
instance, for the formal roles of personnel, and perhaps suggest
that primary care should be more active in screening at-risk groups
in the population rather than passively relying on assumptions about
referral behaviour. Research in this sense is an aspect of
society's self-awareness without which there can be no adaptation,
and there is little reason to believe that social organizations are
any different from biological organisms, in that they either adapt
in time or do not survive.

Any system without a feedback loop runs wild,(68) and medical
and social services are no exception. The crucial place of research
in such systems is illustrated in Figure 9.4. The provision of

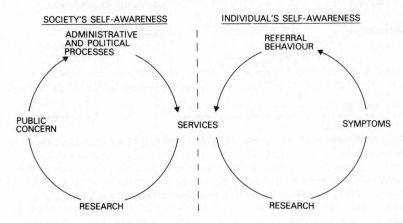

FIGURE 9.4 Research feedback

services is a function of society, whereas their use depends on
individual behaviour. Without research the feedback loops at both
levels are incomplete, so that the system cannot adjust in order
for the two parts to mesh in effectively with the provision of
services. Successful adaptation also requires appropriate attitudes
and the social means of adjustment through administrative and
political processes. But for research to have any effect on the
self-awareness of society the findings must be communicated,
which is the purpose of this book.

REFERENCES

1 Eysenck, H.J. (1958), A Short Questionnaire for the Measurement
   of Two Dimensions of Personality, 'Journal of Applied Psychology',
   42/1, 14-17.
2 Royal College of Physicians, (1971), 'Smoking and Health Now',
   Pitman Medical and Scientific, London.
3 Haddow, A.J. (1967), 'Annual Report', Western Regional Cancer
   Registration Bureau, Glasgow.
4 Hollingsworth, T.H. (1970), 'Migration: A Study Based on
   Scottish Experience', Oliver & Boyd, Edinburgh.
5 Brown, G.W. (1974), 'Stressful Life Events: Their Nature and
   Effects', in Dohrenwend B.S. and Dohrenwend, B.P. (eds), John
   Wiley, New York.
6 Durkheim, E. (1951), 'Suicide - A Study in Sociology', Glencoe
   Press, USA.
7 Kasper, H. (1972), 'Measuring the Labour Market Costs of
   Housing Dislocation', Urban and Regional Studies Discussion
   Papers No.4, University of Glasgow.
8 Boddy, F.A. and Bryden, J.S. (1973), The Computer Experiment,
   'Health Bulletin', 31/3, 166.
9 Berkeley, M. et al. (1972), Computer Compatible Registers for
   General Practice and Research, 'British Journal of Preventive
   and Social Medicine', 26/3, 153-8.
10 Dinwoodie, H.P. (1970), Simple Computer Facilities in General
   Practice, 'Journal of the Royal College of General Practitioners',
   19/94, 269-81.
11 Snaith, A.H. (1971), Health Services and the Computer, 'Health
   Trends', 3/1, 10-11.
12 Bodenham, K.E. and Wellman, F. (1972), 'Foundation for Health
   Service Management', Scientific Control Systems, London.
13 Forbes, J. (1974), 'Studies in Social Science and Planning',
   Scottish Academic Press, Edinburgh.
14 Gruer, R. (1971), Economics of Outpatient Care, 'Lancet', 1,
   390-4.
15 Robertson, I.M.L. (1976), Location of Health Centres in Glasgow.
   Unpublished paper - Department of Town and Regional Planning,
   Glasgow University.
16 Bevan, J.M. and Draper, G.J. (1967), 'Appointment Systems in
   General Practice', Oxford University Press, London.
17 Mayer, J.E., and Timms, N. (1970), 'The Client Speaks',
   Routledge & Kegan Paul, London.
18 Smith, G. (1971), Research Implications of the Seebohm Report,
   'British Journal of Sociology', 22/3, 295-310.
19 Davies, M. (1974), The Current Status of Social Work Research,
   'British Journal of Social Work', 4/3, 283-303.
20 Holson, C.J. and Crayburn Davis, W. (1970), Social Work in a
   Group Medical Practice, 'Psychosomatics', 11/4, 355-7.
21 Bakker, F.R. (1971), An Experiment in Co-ordinating Health Care
   in Rotterdam, 'Huisarts Wetensch', 14/4, 139-51.
22 Confino, R. (1971), Medical-Social Teamwork in the Clinic,
   'Journal of the Royal College of General Practitioners', 21,
   230-40.

23 Richards, K.B. (1972), Health and Social Work - Joint Needs and
    Expectations, 'Health Bulletin', 30/1, 73-8.
24 Watson, D.S. (1972), Value of Social Work in General Practice,
    'Medical Journal of Australia', 1288-91.
25 Vitus, C. (1972), Role of Social Workers, 'South African Medical
    Journal', 46/43, 1646.
26 Westrin, C.G. (1973), Co-operation between Medical and Social
    Services, 'Scand. J. Soc. Med.', 1/3, 115-23.
27 Ratoff, L. et al. (1974), Social Workers and General Practit-
    ioners, 'Social Work Today', 5/16, 497-500.
28 HMSO (1968), 'Royal Commission on Medical Education', London.
29 British Association of Social Workers (1974), Memorandum of
    Evidence to the Committee on the Regulation of the Medical
    Profession, 'Social Work Today', 4/25, 802-3.
30 Bennett, P. et al. (1972), Interprofessional Co-operation,
    'Journal of the Royal College of General Practitioners', 22/122,
    603-9.
31 Lindegard, B. (1973), Social Welfare Care and Patients,
    'Lakartidgingen', 70/3, 194-6.
32 Carstairs, V. (1972), 'Health Services in a Population of
    250,000', Scottish Health Service Studies, No.2, Edinburgh.
33 Scottish Home and Health Department (1971), 'Doctors in an
    Integrated Health Service', HMSO, Edinburgh.
34 James, J.R. (1971), Health Centre Design - A Criticism, 'British
    Medical Journal', 2, 389-93.
35 Rudo, A.B. (1972), Woodside Health Centre - Can I Help You?
    Unpublished paper - Dept. of Community Medicine, Glasgow
    University.
36 Laurie, A. (1969), Health Centre Development, 'Health Bulletin',
    27/3, 46-51.
37 Dixon, P.N. (1971), An Evaluation of Health Centre Practice,
    'Journal of the Royal College of General Practitioners', 21,
    574-80.
38 Parsons, T. (1951), 'The Social System', Routledge & Kegan Paul,
    London.
39 Gordon, G. (1966), 'Role Theory and Illness', College and
    University Press, New Haven, Connecticut.
40 Twaddle, A.C. (1969), Health Decisions and Sick Role Variations,
    'Journal of Health and Social Behaviour', 10/2, 105-14.
41 Petroni, F.A. (1969), The Influence of Age, Sex and Chronicity
    in Perceived Legitimacy to the Sick Role, 'Sociology and Social
    Research', 53/2, 180-93.
42 Petroni, F.A. (1971), Preferred Right to the Sick Role and
    Illness Behaviour, 'Social Science and Medicine', 5, 645-53.
43 Shuval, J.T. et al. (1973), Illness - A Mechanism for Coping
    with Failure, 'Social Science and Medicine', 7, 259-65.
44 Fabrega, H. (1973), Toward a Model of Illness Behaviour,
    'Medical Care', 11, 470-84.
45 Zola, I.K. (1972), Concept of Trouble and Sources of Medical
    Assistance, 'Social Science and Medicine', 6, 673-9.
46 Lamberts, H. (1974), Illness and Problem Behaviour, 'Huisarts
    Wetensch', 17/2, 56-62.
47 Mechanic, D. (1966), The Sociology of Medicine: Viewpoints and
    Perspectives, 'Journal of Health and Human Behaviour', 7/4,
    237-48.

48   Office of Health Economics (1971), 'Prospects in Health', London.
49   Kennedy, D.A. (1973), Perceptions of Illness and Healing, 'Social Science and Medicine', 7, 787-805.
50   Mead, A. (1972), The Future of General Practice in the United Kingdom   A Sociological Diagnosis. Paper at 3rd International Conference on Social Science and Medicine, Elsinore.
51   Office of Health Economics (1974), 'The Work of Primary Medical Care', London.
52   Cullingworth, J.B. (1970), Social Planning in Britain, 'Gerontologist', 10/3, 211-13.
53   Vermost, L. (1974), Counteracting Medical Power: The Sociologists task. Paper at 4th International Conference on Social Science and Medicine, Elsinore.
54   Hart, J.T. (1971), Inverse Care Law, 'Lancet', 1/7696, 405-12.
55   Twaddle, A.C. (1973), Illness and Deviance, 'Social Science and Medicine', 7, 751-62.
56   Pflanz, M. and Rohde, J.J. (1970), Illness: Deviant Behaviour or Conformity? 'Social Science and Medicine', 4, 645-53.
57   Dubos, R. (1959), 'The Mirage of Health', Allen & Unwin, London.
58   Robinson, D. (1971), 'The Process of Becoming Ill', Routledge & Kegan Paul, London.
59   Timms, N. (1970), 'Social Work', Routledge & Kegan Paul, London.
60   Taylor, F.K. (1972), Logical Analysis of Medico-Psychological Concept of Disease, 'Psychological Medicine', 2/1, 7-16.
61   Susser, M. (1973), 'Causal Thinking in the Health Sciences', Oxford University Press, London.
62   Coon, M. and Walsh, J.M. (1974), Developmental Research in Primary Health Care. Paper at 4th International Conference on Social Science and Medicine, Elsinore.
63   Merton, R.K. (1957), 'Social Theory and Social Structure', Glencoe Press, USA.
64   Holtermann, S. (1975), 'Census Indicators of Urban Deprivation', Working Note No.6, Department of the Environment, London.
65   Dahlin, L. and Svanstrom, L. (1973), Population Studies as a Basis for Community Care, 'Lakartidmingen', 70/52, 4845-8.
66   Brozelle, J. (1969), Study on the Health Needs of a Population, 'Bull. Inst. Nat. San. Rech. Med.', 24/3, 613-731.
67   D'Houtaud, A. and Senault, R. (1972), The Importance of Enquiries on Opinions and Attitudes, 'International Journal of Health Education', 15/1, 12-21.
68   Weed, L.L. (1973), Talk on Problem Orientated Medical Records at the Western Informary, Glasgow.

Chapter 10

CONCLUSIONS

This study set out to assess the prevalence of symptoms and referral behaviour in the community, and to relate these to personal charac- teristics, environmental factors, and people's use and perception of services. Inevitably the results describe what was happening in one place at one time, and are limited by the subjective nature of such data. However, the findings have a general relevance to health in the Western world, both for the provision of services such as primary medical care and social work, and for the definition of concepts such as the symptom 'iceberg' and 'trivia'. The main conclusions from the study are summarized below under sub-headings, which reflect the areas covered by the research and the different levels of analysis.

RESPONSE (CHAPTERS 1 AND 2)

1 Almost half the patients drawn from the computer file of a new health centre were not at the address given for them. This was a reflection of the mobility of people in Glasgow partly due to redevelopment.
2 Updating the computer file with changes of address from the health centre, or with additions and deletions from the executive council, had little effect on the accuracy of the file. This was probably because there is no way of registering changes of address for those who are under-utilizers of medical care and frequent movers within an urban area. These tend to be young adults and the survey results were biased accordingly.

SYMPTOMS AND REFERRAL (CHAPTERS 3 AND 4)

3 Eighty-six per cent of all subjects had physical symptoms, of which about one-third were referred for professional advice. Over half such symptoms were not referred at all, with lay referral accounting for 10 per cent.
4 Fifty-one per cent of all adults had mental symptoms of which only 17 per cent were professionally referred. Almost three-quarters

143

of all mental symptoms were not referred at all, with lay referral accounting for 12 per cent.

5 Twenty-four per cent of all children had behavioural symptoms, of which 20 per cent were professionally referred. Nothing was done for 60 per cent of such symptoms, with lay referral accounting for 20 per cent.

6 Twenty-three per cent of all adults had social symptoms, of which half were referred for formal advice. Nothing was done for 41 per cent of such symptoms, with lay referral accounting for 9 per cent.

7 Less than a third of all symptoms were referred for professional or formal advice, the highest proportion being for social symptoms and the least for mental symptoms. Apart from behavioural symptoms in children, lay referral was the least important type of referral.

8 Using the subjective assessments of respondents, the size of the 'iceberg' was 23 per cent of all subjects for medical symptoms, and 4 per cent of all adults for social symptoms.

9 Using the subjective assessments of respondents, medical symptom 'trivia' were referred by 9 per cent of all adults, and social symptom 'trivia' by 3 per cent of all adults.

USE AND PERCEPTION OF MEDICAL SERVICES (CHAPTER 5)

10 Two-thirds of all subjects had visited their doctor during the past year, but only one-quarter had had home visits.

11 The majority of respondents preferred their own doctor as the first source of medical advice, and only 6 per cent made unfavourable comments about their previous experience of doctors and hospitals.

12 Most of those interviewed preferred the health centre to their doctor's previous surgery, and had no comments to make about the health centre, but criticisms of the appointments system were made by 22 per cent of all respondents.

13 Over three-quarters of subjects lived within 20 minutes of the health centre, the majority travelling by bus, but over a quarter came on foot. Eighteen per cent said they had difficulty in seeing or contacting their doctor, almost all due to problems of access to a telephone.

14 About one-third of subjects were on prescribed medicines, and a similar proportion were taking unprescribed medicines. Most of the prescribed medicines resulted from the last visit to a doctor, and most of the unprescribed were obtained from chemists.

15 Almost half those who were married and of child-bearing age said they used no family planning. The pill was the commonest method, and the family doctor the most frequent source of advice and supplies. The majority seemed content with existing facilities.

USE AND PERCEPTION OF SOCIAL WORK   (CHAPTER 6)

16 Less than 10 per cent of respondents had been to a social worker in the past year, and problems with children were the commonest reason for going. Less than 7 per cent of adults who had formally

referred social symptoms found during the survey had done so to
social workers.
17 The majority did not know how to contact a social worker or the
location of a social work department. As many would have gone to
the health centre as to a social work department, in order to contact a social worker.
18 Twenty-two per cent of respondents had had contacts with other
helping agencies during the previous twelve months, mostly with
members of the nursing profession and for physical illness. There
was little indication of any sources of informal neighbourhood
referral.

CORRELATIONS AND MULTIVARIATE ANALYSIS (CHAPTERS 7 AND 8)

19 Over one-quarter of the correlations for measures of symptom
frequency and referral behaviour were significant, but less than a
third of the variance of any of these dependent variables was
accounted for by multivariate analysis.
20 In general, the prevalence of symptoms was highest in the
middle-aged and for females, except that boys had more behavioural
symptoms than girls.
21 There was an overall tendency for the formal referral of medical
symptoms to decrease with age, and to be commoner amongst women.
22 Neuroticism scores increased with symptom frequencies, but not
with the tendency to seek professional advice.
23 Living in high rise flats was associated with an increased
number of mental symptoms, and a tendency formally to refer medical
symptoms and social symptom 'trivia'.
24 Symptom frequencies increased with factors relating to instability such as number of moves for physical symptoms, unemployment
and separation or divorce for mental and social symptoms, and separation from parents for behavioural symptoms in children. Lack of
an active religious allegiance was also associated with increased
prevalence of symptoms.
25 The social problems of a move to better material conditions such
as high flats seemed to be internalized as mental symptoms by the
less perceptive, whereas instabilities relating to housing, unemployment, or marriage were more likely to be externalized as social
symptoms by the more perceptive.
26 In general, factors relating to past medical history and personal
characteristics were more strongly associated with the prevalence of
medical symptoms than factors relating to the environment or to
mobility and stress.
27 The prevalence of social symptoms was more strongly associated
with personal characteristics and measures of mobility and stress,
than with environmental factors or past medical history.
28 Measures of present health seemed to be more important determinants of patterns of referral than perceptions of services,
assessments of which tended to reflect the consequences rather than
the causes of referral behaviour.

IMPLICATIONS (CHAPTER 9)

29   In view of the rate of intra-urban mobility, accurate population
data as a basis for the provision of services may only be possible
through a formal system of address registration.
30   The present location of doctors' surgeries might be a more
realistic and feasible criterion for siting health centres than the
postulated projections of a highly mobile population.
31   Appointments systems require greater flexibility especially
when first introduced.
32   In view of the size of the symptom 'iceberg' and its apparent
relationship to personality, official campaigns to discourage people
from troubling their doctor may be misplaced.
33   There is a need for feedback from consumers not only as a base
line for the provision of new services, but as a continual process
of evaluation and adjustment.
34   The objectives of social work require clarification and
evaluation.
35   The medical and social work professions need a better understanding of each other, and this might best be achieved by shared
experience in training.
36   Most of the causes of physical, mental, and social malaise,
which are amenable to change, lie largely outside the practical
remits of the caring professions.
37   There is a place in primary medical care for more active
screening of at-risk groups in the population.
38   Medical and social services of first contact should be developed
as a coherent whole from the basis of existing referral patterns.
39   The concept of adaptation provides a better conceptual framework
for understanding illness and referral behaviour than theories based
on the sick role or deviance.
40   Successful adaptation, whether for individuals or society,
requires self-awareness and the ability to adjust, for which the
continual feedback of information is essential.

APPENDIX I

THE QUESTIONNAIRE

The sheets were stapled inside the top of the right-hand cover of a simple cardboard folder, so that the pages could be turned over like a 'memo pad'. The two pages of symptom grading scales were attached to the left-hand cover for ease of reference.

The answers to questions were coded directly in boxes down the right-hand margins of the pages, except those questions marked with an asterisk which were coded afterwards (post-coded). The coding boxes were numbered for 80 column cards, so that the information could be transferred directly from the questionnaires to punched cards.

CONFIDENTIAL

SURVEY OF SYMPTOMS AND SYMPTOM BEHAVIOUR IN GLASGOW

Interviewer code
Number of subject
*Locality code
*Practice
Date of interview   Day
                                                              Month
Time of commencing interview

Age in years

Sex
0   Not known
1   Male
2   Female

Marital status
0   Not known
1   Single
2   Married
3   Separated or divorced

147

4 Widow or widower
5 Other (specify)

Employment status of subject
0 Not known
1 Employed, full-time
2 Employed, part-time
3 Unemployed, due to illness
4 Unemployed, not due to illness
5 Child of 15 yrs and under
6 Student of 16 yrs and over if full-time
7 Housewife
8 Retired
9 Other

*Occupation
Present or last full-time occupation: (Father's if child or student, husband's if housewife; own if widowed, separated, or divorced.)
(specify)
(Note if unemployed or retired)
    0 Not known
    1 Registrar General's Social Class 1
    2   "   "   "   "   2
    3   "   "   "   "   3a
    4   "   "   "   "   3b
    5   "   "   "   "   4
    6   "   "   "   "   5
    7 None

Education
0 Not known
1 None - under 5 years old
2 At school - 5 to 15 years old
3 Left school at 13 years or under
4 Left school at 14 years
5 Left school at 15 years
6 Stayed or staying for 1 year of full-time education
7 Stayed or staying for 2 years of full-time education
8 Stayed or staying for 3 years of full-time education
9 Stayed or staying for 4 or more years of full-time education
   (Specify if > 4)

Religion
0 Not known
1 None/Atheist/Agnostic
2 Church of Scotland Active (Attend at least once a month)
3 Church of Scotland Passive (Attend less than once a month)
4 Other Protestant Denomination Active
5 Other Protestant Denomination Passive
6 Roman Catholic   Active
7 Roman Catholic   Passive
8 Other (specify)   Active
9 Other (specify)   Passive

Relationship to housing tenure
O   Not known
1   Owner-occupier or spouse of
2   Tenant or spouse of - Corporation
3   Tenant or spouse of - other owner
4   Relative of owner-occupier
5   Relative of Corporation tenant
6   Relative of other tenant
7   Institution
8   Other (specify)

When was the dwelling built?
O   Not known
1   Pre-1914
2   1914-44
3   Post 1944

What type of dwelling is it?
O   Not known
1   Detached or semi-detached house
2   Terraced house
    Flat or maisonette in low rise block or tenement:
3   Basement, Ground or 1st floor
4   2nd, 3rd, or 4th floor
    Flat or maisonette in high rise block with lift:
5   Basement, Ground, or 1st floor
6   2nd, 3rd, or 4th floor
7   5th to 10th floor
8   11th floor or over
9   Other (specify)

Number of rooms in dwelling (excluding bathroom, toilet, passage,
staircase, kitchen < 6 feet across, and cupboards)
O   Not known
1-8 Number of rooms
9   Nine or more rooms

Number of occupants normally resident in household (including
relatives, children, babies, and lodgers)
O   Not known
1-8 Number of occupants
9   Nine or more occupants

Water closet
O   Not known
1   Inside dwelling for own use
2   Outside dwelling for own use
3   Outside dwelling, shared
4   None
5   Other

Hot water and fixed bath or shower
O   Not known
1   Both hot water and fixed bath or shower present

2 Hot water present but no fixed bath or shower
3 Fixed bath or shower present, but no hot water
4 Neither hot water nor fixed bath or shower present
5 Other

Length of residence in present dwelling, in years

Length of registration with present GP, in years

Location of previous residence before the present one
0 Not known
1 No previous residence
2 In the City of Glasgow
3 Outside the City of Glasgow but within the Clyde Valley
   conurbation (Renfrew, Lanark, Dunbartonshire)
4 Elsewhere in Scotland
5 England or Wales
6 Ireland (North or South)
7 Other (specify)
(Specify if same street or staircase for 2 and 3)

Mother's residence at time of birth of subject
0 Not known
1 Mother resident at present address (or staircase)
2 Mother resident elsewhere in the City of Glasgow
3 Mother resident outside the City of Glasgow but within the
   Clyde Valley conurbation (Renfrew, Lanark, Dunbartonshire)
4 Elsewhere in Scotland
5 England or Wales
6 Ireland (North or South)
7 Other (specify)
(Specify if same street for 2 and 3)

Main place of upbringing and schooling to 15 years
0 Not known
1 Present address (or staircase)
2 Elsewhere in the City of Glasgow
3 Outside the City of Glasgow but within the Clyde Valley
   conurbation (Renfrew, Lanark, Dunbartonshire)
4 Elsewhere in Scotland
5 England or Wales
6 Ireland (North or South)
7 Other (specify)
(Specify if same street for 2 and 3)

How many times have you changed your place of permanent residence?
(i.e. more than 6 months' stay)
00 Not known or none
1-99 Number of times   (Code number)

On how many occasions during the past week have you seen any close
relative or relatives? (apart from those in same household)
0 Not known
1 0

2   1
3   2 or 3
4   4 to 6
5   7 or more
Specify relative(s)

PAST MEDICAL HISTORY

Have you ever had any serious illnesses, accidents, or operations?
(Exclude coughs and colds, sprains and bruises, childhood illnesses
such as measles, and normal childbirth)
Nature of illness, accident, or operation   Age at time

                                    (Code number - 9 if 9 or more)

How many times have you been in hospital?
Short term (at least one night, and less than 6 months)
                                    (Code number - 9 if 9 or more)
Long term (for periods of 6 months or more)
                                    (Code number - 9 if 9 or more)

*How would you describe your experience of doctors and hospitals?
(If the subject is a child, specify whether comments are for the
child or for the adult answering for the child)

How would you describe your present state of health?
O   Not known
1   Perfect
2   Good
3   Fair
4   Poor
5   Very poor

Have you any illnesses or disabilities at the moment?
Nature of illness or disability   Duration

                                    (Code number - 9 if 9 or more)

SYMPTOM CHECK LIST

Please could you tell me if you have noticed any of the following things about yourself during the past two weeks or at the moment:

Feeling more tired than usual or generally run-down
0   Not known
1   No
2   Yes - more tired than usual
3   Yes - generally run-down
4   Yes - 2 and 3

A change in your weight, e.g.:
0   Not known
1   No
2   Yes - Loss of weight (exclude deliberate dieting)
3   Yes - Gain in weight (exclude pregnancy)

Fever, or unusual sweating or flushing
0   Not known
1   No
2   Yes - Fever
3   Yes - Unusual sweating
4   Yes - Unusual flushing
5   Yes - 2 and 3
6   Yes - 3 and 4
7   Yes - 2 and 4
8   Yes - 2, 3, and 4

Trouble with skin, e.g.:
0   Not known
1   No
2   Yes - Rash or irritation
3   Yes - Sores or ulcers
4   Yes - Boils or other (specify)
5   Yes - 2 and 3
6   Yes - 3 and 4
7   Yes - 2 and 4
8   Yes, 2, 3, and 4

Trouble with hair, e.g.:
0   Not known
1   No
2   Yes - Loss of hair
3   Yes - Superfluous hair
4   Yes - Dandruff
5   Yes - 2 and 3
6   Yes - 3 and 4
7   Yes - 2 and 4
8   Yes - 2, 3, and 4

Lumps under skin, e.g.:
        0   Not known
        1   No

```
          2  Yes - Lumps or swollen glands (other than in breast)
          3  Yes - Swellings such as a rupture
(w ⩾ 16)  4  Yes - Lumps in breast
          5  Yes - 2 and 3
(w ⩾ 16)  6  Yes - 3 and 4
(w ⩾ 16)  7  Yes - 2 and 4
(w ⩾ 16)  8  Yes - 2, 3, and 4
```

Change of colour in skin or in whites of the eyes, e.g.:
0 Not known
1 No
2 Yes - Paler than usual
3 Yes - Yellower than usual
4 Yes - Other discolouration such as bruising
5 Yes - 2 and 3
6 Yes - 3 and 4
7 Yes - 2 and 4
8 Yes - 2, 3, and 4

Feeling more thirsty than usual, or cold apart from the weather:
0 Not known
1 No
2 Yes - More thirsty than usual
3 Yes - More cold, apart from the weather
4 Yes - 2 and 3

Change of appetite
0 Not known
1 No
2 Yes - Loss of appetite
3 Yes - Gain of appetite, or feeling hungry

Trouble with teeth, or difficulty in eating or swallowing, e.g.:
0 Not known
1 No
2 Yes - Trouble with teeth
3 Yes - Difficulty in eating because of mouth or gums
4 Yes - Difficulty in swallowing because of trouble in throat
        (or oesophagus)
5 Yes - 2 and 3
6 Yes - 3 and 4
7 Yes - 2 and 4
8 Yes - 2, 3, and 4

Nausea or vomiting, e.g.:
```
      0  Not known
      1  No
      2  Yes - Nausea or feeling like vomiting
      3  Yes - Retching without bringing up food (include phlegm or
             watery stuff)
      4  Yes - Vomiting up food or drink
(D)   5  Yes - Vomiting up blood which had not been swallowed
```

Heartburn or indigestion, e.g.:
0 Not known
1 No
2 Yes - Heartburn (burning feeling behind sternum associated with
         food)
3 Yes - Indigestion (upper abdominal pain or discomfort associated
         with food)
4 Yes - 2 and 3

Other abdominal or tummy pains (other than period pains) or trouble
with bowels, e.g.:
0 Not known
1 No
2 Yes - Pains in abdomen or tummy
3 Yes - Diarrhoea (more loose or frequent than usual)
4 Yes - Constipation (harder or less frequent than usual)
5 Yes - 2 and 3
6 Yes - 3 and 4
7 Yes - 2 and 4
8 Yes - 2, 3, and 4

Trouble when opening bowels, e.g.:
0 Not known
1 No
2 Yes - Pain on defaecation
3 Yes - Red blood on stool or paper
4 Yes - 2 and 3

Difficulty or discomfort in passing water (urine) e.g.:
0 Not known
1 No
2 Yes - More difficult than usual (poor stream or dribbling)
3 Yes - Discomfort such as pain or burning
4 Yes - 2 and 3

Passing water (urine) more often than usual, e.g.:
0 Not known
1 No
2 Yes - More frequently during the day
3 Yes - More frequently at night
4 Yes - 2 and 3

(A $\geqslant$ 11) Trouble with water (urine) coming away too quickly, e.g.:
0 Not known
1 No
2 Yes - Have to run to toilet
3 Yes - Leaks when straining, coughing, or laughing
4 Yes - 2 and 3

Unusual colour or smell about water (urine), e.g.:
     0 Not known
     1 No
     2 Yes - Strong smell

(D) 3   Yes - Reddish/brown discolouration
(D) 4   Yes - 2 and 3

(A ⩾ 16) Pain or swelling in private parts (men), or front passage
(women), e.g.:
0   Not known
1   No
2   Yes - Pain (include on intercourse if married)
3   Yes - Swelling (include prolapse or bulging down below, for
          women)
4   Yes - 2 and 3

(A ⩾ 16) Discharge or irritation in private parts (men), or front
passage (women), e.g.:
0   Not known
1   No
2   Yes - Discharge (if unusual for women)
3   Yes - Irritation
4   Yes - 2 and 3

(W ⩾ 16) Trouble with periods, e.g.
     0   Not known
     1   No
     2   Yes - Pain with last period
     3   Yes - Unusually heavy last period
(D) 4   Yes - Bleeding between periods, or any bleeding if post-
              menopausal
     5   Yes - 2 and 3
(D) 6   Yes - 3 and 4
(D) 7   Yes - 2 and 4
(D) 8   Yes - 2, 3, and 4

(W ⩾ 16) Irregularity or absence of period if pre-menopausal, e.g.:
0   Not known
1   No
2   Yes - Irregularity of periods
3   Yes - Absence of periods (probably) not pregnant
4   Yes - Absence of periods (probably) pregnant

(W ⩾ 16) Trouble with pregnancy (if pregnant), e.g.:
0   Not known
1   No
2   Yes - Morning sickness
3   Yes - Pain or bleeding
4   Yes - Other (specify)
5   Yes - 2 and 3
6   Yes - 3 and 4
7   Yes - 2 and 4
8   Yes - 2, 3, and 4
(If symptom associated with pregnancy by the subject, include here
and delete from elsewhere)

Trouble with your nose, e.g.:
0   Not known
1   No
2   Yes - Stuffy or runny nose, or catarrh at the back of the nose
3   Yes - Nose bleeds
4   Yes - 2 and 3

Trouble with your throat or voice, e.g.:
0   Not known
1   No
2   Yes - Sore throats
3   Yes - Hoarseness or loss of voice (including laryngitis)
4   Yes - Other (specify)
5   Yes - 2 and 3
6   Yes - 3 and 4
7   Yes - 2 and 4
8   Yes - 2, 3, and 4

Cough (ask both questions as indicated)
0   Not known
1   No
2   Yes - Do you have a cough now, or during the past 2 weeks?
3   Yes - Do you usually cough first thing on getting up (include
            coughing with first smoke or on first going out of doors;
            exclude clearing throat or occasional cough)?
4   Yes - 2 and 3

Phlegm (ask both questions as indicated)
0   Not known
1   No
2   Yes - Do you bring up phlegm now, or during the past 2 weeks?
3   Yes - Do you usually bring up phlegm first thing on getting up
            (include phlegm with first smoke or on first going out of
            doors, and swallowed phlegm; exclude phlegm from nose or
            single episode of bringing up phlegm)?
4   Yes - 2 and 3

Wheezing or coughing up blood, e.g.:
      0   Not known
      1   No
      2   Yes - Chest sounding wheezy and whistling
      3   Yes - Attacks of shortness of breath with wheezing
(D)   4   Yes - Coughing up blood which had not been swallowed
      5   Yes - 2 and 3
(D)   6   Yes - 3 and 4
(D)   7   Yes - 2 and 4
(D)   8   Yes - 2, 3, and 4

Shortness of breath, e.g.:
0   Not known
1   No
2   Yes - When hurrying on level ground or walking up slight hill
3   Yes - When walking with people of own age on level ground
4   Yes - Have to stop for breath when walking at own pace on level
            ground

5 Yes - When washing or dressing
6 Yes - When sitting quietly
(Code highest number)

Attacks of palpitations or breathlessness, e.g.:
0 Not known
1 No
2 Yes - Attacks of palpitations when heart beats fast for no
             apparent reason
3 Yes - Attacks of breathlessness when lying down
4 Yes - Sudden attacks of breathlessness when lying down at night
5 Yes - 2 and 3
6 Yes - 3 and 4
7 Yes - 2 and 4
8 Yes - 2, 3, and 4

Ankle swelling or varicose veins
0 Not known
1 No
2 Yes - Ankle swelling in both ankles
3 Yes - Varicose veins
4 Yes - 2 and 3

Pain or discomfort in chest which may go to arm (especially the left),
e.g.:
0 Not known
1 No
2 Yes - Comes on when walking and goes in 10 minutes or less if
             stop or slow down
3 Yes - Severe pain across front of chest which lasts for half an
             hour or more
4 Yes - 2 and 3
5 Yes - Other pain or discomfort in chest (specify)

Pain in calf of either leg, e.g.:
0 Not known
1 No
2 Yes - Comes on when standing still or sitting
3 Yes - Comes on only when walking, and goes in 10 minutes or less
             if stand still
4 Yes - 2 and 3
5 Yes - Other pain in calf of either leg (e.g. cramps)
             (specify)

Have you had any injuries during the past two weeks, e.g.:
0 Not known
1 No
2 Yes - burn
3 Yes - Other minor injury or accident such as fall with bruising
4 Yes - Other more serious injury or accident such as fall with
             broken bone
5 Yes - 2 and 3
6 Yes - 3 and 4
7 Yes - 2 and 4

8 Yes - 2, 3, and 4
(If symptom associated with injury sustained during past 2 weeks,
code here and delete from elsewhere)

Trouble with joints, e.g.:
0 Not known
1 No
2 Yes - Pain, swelling, tenderness, or redness in small joints of
         hands or feet
3 Yes - Pain, swelling, tenderness, or redness in large joints
4 Yes - Morning stiffness
5 Yes - 2 and 3
6 Yes - 3 and 4
7 Yes - 2 and 4
8 Yes - 2, 3, and 4

Pain in spine or large bones, e.g.:
0 Not known
1 No
2 Yes - Low back pain
3 Yes - Pain elsewhere in spine
4 Yes - Pain in large bones (e.g. arms, legs, pelvis)
         (specify)
5 Yes - 2 and 3
6 Yes - 3 and 4
7 Yes - 2 and 4
8 Yes - 2, 3, and 4

Trouble with feet, e.g.:
0 Not known
1 No
2 Yes - Bunions, corns, or callosities
3 Yes - Ingrowing toenails
4 Yes - Flat feet or other (specify)
5 Yes - 2 and 3
6 Yes - 3 and 4
7 Yes - 2 and 4
8 Yes - 2, 3, and 4

Loss of consciousness (exclude anaesthetics) or convulsions, e.g.:
0 Not known
1 No
2 Yes - Loss of consciousness or black-outs
3 Yes - Convulsions or fits
4 Yes - 2 and 3

Headaches or dizziness, or feeling more irritable and jumpy than
usual, e.g.:
0 Not known
1 No
2 Yes - Headaches (include migraine)
3 Yes - Spells of dizziness or vertigo
4 Yes - Feeling more irritable and jumpy than usual
5 Yes - 2 and 3

6 Yes - 3 and 4
7 Yes - 2 and 4
8 Yes - 2, 3, and 4

Facial pain, loss of speech or balance, e.g.:
0 Not known
1 No
2 Yes - Pain in face for no apparent reason (exclude teeth)
3 Yes - Loss of power of speech
4 Yes - Loss of ability to balance on feet
5 Yes - 2 and 3
6 Yes - 3 and 4
7 Yes - 2 and 4
8 Yes - 2, 3, and 4

Trouble with ears, e.g.:
0 Not known
1 No
2 Yes - Pain, irritation, or wax in ears
3 Yes - Difficulty in hearing
4 Yes - Ringing or buzzing in ears
5 Yes - 2 and 3
6 Yes - 3 and 4
7 Yes - 2 and 4
8 Yes - 2, 3, and 4

Trouble with eyes, e.g.:
0 Not known
1 No
2 Yes - Pain, irritation, or watering of eyes (specify)
3 Yes - Difficulty in seeing (with glasses if present)
4 Yes - Loss of sight in one or both eyes
5 Yes - 2 and 3
6 Yes - 3 and 4
7 Yes - 2 and 4
8 Yes - 2, 3, and 4

Loss of power in limbs, e.g.:
0 Not known
1 No
2 Yes - Loss of power in upper limb(s) (include hands)
3 Yes - Loss of power in lower limb(s) (include feet)
4 Yes - 2 and 3

Loss of feeling or alteration of sensation in limbs, e.g.:
0 Not known
1 No
2 Yes - Loss of feeling, tingling or numbness in upper limb(s)
         (include hands)
3 Yes - Loss of feeling, tingling or numbness in lower limb(s)
         (include feet)
4 Yes - 2 and 3

THE FOLLOWING QUESTIONS ARE FOR ADULTS OF 16 YEARS AND OVER ONLY

Anxiety, fears, or loneliness, e.g.:
0   Not known
1   No
2   Yes - Feeling anxious at times without knowing the reason
3   Yes - Afraid of being in a wide open space or enclosed space
4   Yes - Feeling lonely
5   Yes - 2 and 3
6   Yes - 3 and 4
7   Yes - 2 and 4
8   Yes - 2, 3, and 4

Sleeplessness, e.g.:
0   Not known
1   No
2   Yes - Difficulty in getting off to sleep without sleeping pills
3   Yes - Waking in the early hours and being unable to get off to
          sleep again if you don't have sleeping pills
4   Yes - 2 and 3

Loss of interest in things, e.g.:
0   Not known
1   No
2   Yes - Losing interest in almost everything
3   Yes - Finding it difficult to concentrate
4   Yes - Being slower in everything you do
5   Yes - 2 and 3
6   Yes - 3 and 4
7   Yes - 2 and 4
8   Yes - 2, 3, and 4

Worries about other people, e.g.:
0   Not known
1   No
2   Yes - People talking about you and criticizing you through no
          fault of your own
3   Yes - People trying to harm you through no fault of your own
4   Yes - 2 and 3

Are you bothered by periods of excitability? e.g.:
0   Not known
1   No
2   Yes - Times when exciting new ideas and schemes occur to you one
          after the other
3   Yes - Being so cheerful that you want to laugh and joke with
          everyone
4   Yes - 2 and 3

Are you bothered by worries about doing things exactly right, e.g.:
0   Not known
1   No
2   Yes - Feeling you have to check things again and again - like
          turning off taps or lights, shutting windows at night, etc.
          - although you know there is really no need to

3 Yes - Having an uneasy feeling if you don't do something in a
          certain order, or a certain number of times
4 Yes - 2 and 3

Feeling puzzled, e.g.:
O Not known
1 No
2 Yes - Feeling puzzled, as if something had gone wrong either with
          you or with the world, without knowing just what it is
3 Yes - Hearing voices without knowing where they come from
4 Yes - 2 and 3

Feeling low in spirits, e.g.:
O Not known
1 No
2 Yes - Being so low in spirits that you just sit for hours on end
3 Yes - Going to bed feeling you wouldn't care if you never woke up
4 Yes - 2 and 3

CIGARETTE SMOKING (ADULTS ONLY)

Have you ever smoked cigarettes regularly?
O Not known
1 No, never
2 Yes - In the past but not now, and did not inhale
3 Yes - In the past but not now, and inhaled
4 Yes - Now, but do not inhale
5 Yes - Now, and inhale

If you used to smoke but don't now, how long is it since you gave
it up?
O Not known
1 Not relevant as smoke now
2 Less than 1 year
3 1 - 5 years
4 6 - 10 years
5 10 - 20 years
6 20 - 40 years
7 > 40 years

How many cigarettes do you, or did you, smoke a day?

THE FOLLOWING QUESTIONS ARE TO BE ASKED ABOUT CHILDREN OF 15 YEARS
AND UNDER ONLY

(All ages of 15 or less)   Do you think he or she is more difficult
to manage than others of the same age? e.g.:
O Not known
1 No
2 Yes - Cries a lot or continually whining
3 Yes - Has real temper tantrums
4 Yes - Disobedient and/or sulky
5 Yes - 2 and 3

6 Yes - 3 and 4
7 Yes - 2 and 4
8 Yes - 2, 3, and 4

(All ages of 15 or less) Is there any other way in which he or she
is more difficult to manage than others of the same age?
0 Not known
1 No
2 Yes (specify)

(0 to 1 years only) Not alert or not smiling, e.g.:
        0 Not known, or wrong age
        1 No
        2 Yes - Not as alert as usual, or compared to other
            babies of same age
($\geqslant$ 2/12) 3 Yes - Not smiling at mother or equivalent (if more than
            2 months old only)
        4 Yes - 2 and 3

(1 year only) Difficulty in sitting up on own or crawling
0 Not known, or wrong age
1 No
2 Yes - Difficulty in sitting up
3 Yes - Difficulty in crawling
4 Yes - 2 and 3

(2 years only) Difficulty in standing or walking on own
0 Not known, or wrong age
1 No
2 Yes - Difficulty in standing on own
3 Yes - Difficulty in walking on own
4 Yes - 2 and 3

(3-5 years only) Difficulty in playing with other children, e.g.:
0 Not known, or wrong age
1 No
2 Yes - Does not play well with other children of the same age
       because always fighting or quarrelling
3 Yes - Does not play well with other children of the same age
       because shy and does not have friends of same age
4 Yes - Other (specify)
5 Yes - 2 and 3
6 Yes - 3 and 4
7 Yes - 2 and 4
8 Yes - 2, 3, and 4

(3-5 years only) Difficulty with talking or sleeping, e.g.:
0 Not known, or wrong age
1 No
2 Yes - Does not talk as well as he or she should for age
3 Yes - Restless in sleep - tosses and turns - wakes in the night -
       has frightening dreams
4 Yes - Other (specify)
5 Yes - 2 and 3
6 Yes - 3 and 4

7 Yes - 2 and 4
8 Yes - 2, 3, and 4

(6-10 years inclusive) Difficulty with friends or at school, e.g.:
0 Not known, or wrong age
1 No
2 Yes - Difficulty in making and keeping friends
3 Yes - Difficulty in school work or learning to read compared
          with other children of same age
4 Yes - Other (specify)
5 Yes - 2 and 3
6 Yes - 3 and 4
7 Yes - 2 and 4
8 Yes - 2, 3, and 4

(6-10 years inclusive) Bed-wetting, e.g.:
0 Not known, or wrong age
1 No
2 Yes - Occasionally
3 Yes - Sometimes
4 Yes - Frequently, on most nights

(11-15 years inclusive) Difficulty with friends or at school, e.g.:
0 Not known, or wrong age
1 No
2 Yes - Difficulty in making and keeping friends
3 Yes - Difficulty with school work compared with children of
          same age
4 Yes - Other (specify)
5 Yes - 2 and 3
6 Yes - 3 and 4
7 Yes - 2 and 4
8 Yes - 2, 3, and 4

(11-15 years inclusive) Getting into trouble, e.g.:
0 Not known, or wrong age
1 No
2 Yes - Gets into trouble a lot at school (include truancy)
3 Yes - Gets into trouble outside school (police, probation,
          children's panels, etc.)
4 Yes - Other (specify)
5 Yes - 2 and 3
6 Yes - 3 and 4
7 Yes - 2 and 4
8 Yes - 2, 3, and 4

WHO IS BEING INTERVIEWED ABOUT THE CHILD?

0 Not known
1 Parent
2 Grandparent
3 Brother or sister
4 Uncle or aunt
5 Cousin

6   Foster parent
7   Guardian
8   Other (specify)

Age in years

Sex
0   Not known
1   Male
2   Female

THE FOLLOWING QUESTIONS ARE FOR ADULTS OR 16 YEARS AND OVER ONLY

(Those with children only) Are there are difficulties with children
or teenagers which have been troubling you during the past two weeks?
0   Not known
1   No
2   Yes - caused slight worry and/or inconvenience
3   Yes - caused moderate worry and/or inconvenience
4   Yes - caused a lot of worry and/or inconvenience

*Nature of trouble, and duration

*Who involved? (relationship, age, sex)

*What have you done about it?

*Why?

(All adults ≥ 16) Are there any difficulties with other members of
the family or relatives (other than children and teenagers) which
have been troubling you during the past two weeks?
0   Not known
1   No
2   Yes - caused slight worry and/or inconvenience
3   Yes - caused moderate worry and/or inconvenience
4   Yes - caused a lot of worry and/or inconvenience

*Nature of trouble, and duration?

*Who involved? (relationship, age, sex)

*What have you done about it?

*Why?

(All adults ≥ 16) Are there any financial difficulties which have
been troubling you during the past two weeks?
0   Not known
1   No
2   Yes - caused slight worry and/or inconvenience
3   Yes - caused moderate worry and/or inconvenience
4   Yes - caused a lot of worry and/or inconvenience

*Nature of problem and duration?

*What have you done about it?

*Why?

(All adults ≥ 16) Are there any other difficulties or problems with day-to-day life which have been troubling you during the past two weeks?
0   Not known
1   No
2   Yes - caused slight worry and/or inconvenience
3   Yes - caused moderate worry and/or inconvenience
4   Yes - caused a lot of worry and/or inconvenience

*Nature of problem(s), and duration?

*What have you done about it or them?

*Why?

(Specify below if several difficulties and problems, and not sufficient space above)

THE FOLLOWING TO BE SELF-COMPLETED BY ALL THOSE BEING INTERVIEWED, INCLUDING THOSE ANSWERING FOR CHILDREN

*The answers to be completed by the subject
Here are some questions regarding the way you behave, feel, or act. Try to decide whether 'Yes' or 'No' represents your usual way of acting or feeling, and then put a circle round the 'Yes' or 'No'. Work quickly, and don't spend too much time over any one question. Give your first reaction, and not the result after long thought. There are no right and wrong answers.

Do you like doing things where you have to act quickly?	Yes	No
Do you sometimes feel happy, sometimes depressed, without any apparent reason?	Yes	No
Does your mind often wander while you are trying to concentrate?	Yes	No
When you make new friends do you usually make the first move?	Yes	No
Are you quick and sure in your actions?	Yes	No
Are you often lost in thought?	Yes	No
Are you sometimes bubbling over with energy and sometimes very sluggish?	Yes	No
Are you a lively person?	Yes	No
Would you be very unhappy if you were prevented from seeing and talking to a lot of people?	Yes	No
Do you sometimes sulk?	Yes	No
Does your mood often go up and down, either with or without reason?	Yes	No
Do you prefer doing something, rather than thinking about how to do it?	Yes	No

Self-completed intelligence test for all those being interviewed,
including those answering for children. Eight questions derived
from Cattell 16 Personality Factor - Form C.

FROM HERE ON THE QUESTIONS ARE TO BE ASKED OF ALL THOSE BEING
INTERVIEWED, INCLUDING THOSE ANSWERING FOR CHILDREN

Have you (or the child) seen your GP, partner, or locum in his
surgery during the past twelve months?
0   Not known
1   No
2   Yes - Once
3   Yes - 2 or 3 times
4   Yes - 4 to 6 times
5   Yes - 7 to 12 times
6   Yes - 13 or more times (i.e., more than once a month)

Have you (or the child) seen your GP, partner, or locum at your home
during the past twelve months?
0   Not known
1   No
2   Yes - Once
3   Yes - 2 or 3 times
4   Yes - 4 to 6 times
5   Yes - 7 to 12 times
6   Yes - 13 or more times (i.e., more than once a month)

Do you think the Health Centre is an improvement on your doctor's
previous surgery?
0   Not known
1   No
2   Yes
3   Never been to doctor's previous surgery
4   Never been to Health Centre
5   Never been to either
6   Don't know

*Do you think the Health Centre arrangements could be improved in
any way? (specify)

Have you (or the child) seen a social worker during the past twelve
months?
0   Not known
1   No
2   Yes - Once
3   Yes - 2 or 3 times
4   Yes - 4 to 6 times
5   Yes - 7 to 12 times
6   Yes - 13 or more times (i.e., more than once a month)

*What were you seeing the social worker for?   (specify)

*What sort of problems do you think social workers deal with?
 (specify)

*Do you know anyone else who has been to a social worker?
 (specify - who, and for what reason)

*Have you had any contacts with other helping agencies during the
 past twelve months?
 Such as: nurses, health visitors, child guidance, home helps
 (specify)
*(reasons for contact)

How do you, or would you, contact your doctor if you wanted to?
0 Not known
1 Don't know
2 Attend health centre without appointment
3 Attend health centre to make an appointment
4 Telephone doctor directly
5 Telephone health centre for appointment
6 Write to doctor or health centre for appointment
7 Get friend or relative to telephone
8 Get friend or relative to call and make appointment
9 Other (specify)

*Do you have any difficulty in seeing or contacting your doctor or
 the health centre? (specify)
 (e.g. access to a telephone)

How do you travel from your home to the Woodside Health Centre?
0 Not known
1 Don't know
2 Walk
3 Bus
4 Train
5 Car or taxi
6 Other (specify)
7 Combination of 3, 4, 5, or 6

Travelling this way, how long does it take you to get from your
home to the Woodside Health Centre?
Code in minutes

How do you, or would you, contact a social worker?
0 Not known
1 Don't know
2 Call at Social Work Department
3 Ring up Social Work Department
4 Write to Social Work Department
5 Ask friend or relative
6 Ask at health centre
7 Ask other formal agency (specify)
8 Other (specify)

*Where is the nearest Social Work Department?
 (Comment on reply, i.e. do they really know?)

MEDICAL KNOWLEDGE TEST

Which, if either, is most likely to cause ill health - pipe smoking
or cigarette smoking?
(Correct answer - cigarette smoking - scores 1)   Score

Which, if either, is most likely to be serious - a nose
bleed, or coughing up blood which had not been swallowed?
(Correct answer - coughing up blood - scores 1)   Score

Which, if any, of the following may be partly caused by
smoking cigarettes?
Lung Cancer   (Yes)
Bronchitis   (Yes)
Heart Disease (Yes)
(Correct answer - all three - scores 3)   Score

Which, if any, of the following can you catch from someone else?
Diabetes   (No)
Polio   (Yes)
Tuberculosis (Yes)
Anaemia   (No)
(Correct answer - as above - scores 4)   Score

Code total score out of 9

*Is there anyone in your neighbourhood to whom lots of people from
 round about go for advice with problems?
 (specify and comment)

If you are in doubt about a symptom, is it better to wait and see
how it develops, or take it straight to the doctor?
0 Not known
1 Don't know
2 Wait and see how it develops
3 Take it straight to the doctor
4 Other (specify)

Do you think that for many complaints, home remedies are just as
good as anything the doctor can give you?
0 Not known
1 Don't know
2 No
3 Yes
4 About the same
5 Depends on the complaint

When you first feel there is something you would like to see a
doctor about, who would you want to see first?
0 Not known
1 Own doctor
2 Either own doctor or one of his partners
3 Any doctor at the health centre
4 A specialist
5 Don't mind - any doctor
6 Don't know

MEDICINES

Are you, or the child, taking any medicines at the moment (or during the past two weeks) which were prescribed by your doctor?
0   Not known
1   No
2   Yes - Prescribed for subject when last saw doctor
3   Yes - Repeat prescription for subject without seeing doctor
4   Yes - Prescribed for someone other than subject
5   Yes - 2 and 3
6   Yes - 3 and 4
7   Yes - 2 and 4
8   Yes - 2, 3, and 4

*What prescribed medicines? (specify)

Are you, or the child, taking any medicines at the moment (or during the past two weeks) which were not prescribed by a doctor?
0   Not known
1   No
2   Yes - Bought from a chemist
3   Yes - Obtained from other source (specify)

*What unprescribed medicines? (specify)
 (prompt: Aspirins, Askits, etc.)

FAMILY PLANNING

(For all married people, whether answering for self or for child, providing the wife is of child-bearing age)

What method of contraception do you use?
0   Not known or not applicable
1   None
2   Pill
3   Cap
4   Coil
5   Sheath
6   Chemicals on own
7   Husband withdraws
8   Safe period
9   Other (specify)

*Where have you got advice about contraception?
 (specify)

*Where do you obtain contraceptive supplies?
 (specify)

*Do you think there are adequate facilities for obtaining advice about family planning and contraceptive supplies?
0   Not known
1   Yes
2   No (comment)

*Are there any other personal matters about which you would have
liked some advice during the past two weeks?
O Not known
1 No
2 Yes (specify)

THANK YOU VERY MUCH FOR YOUR HELP

*Are there any comments you would like to make about the interview?
 (e.g., Being too long, too personal, etc.)

Time of finishing interview
Length of interview in minutes

Others present during all or most of the interview
(specify)
O Not known
1 Subject alone
2 Parent(s)
3 Brother(s) or sister(s)
4 Husband or wife
5 Subject's child or children
6 Other (specify)
7 Combination of above

INTERVIEWER'S COMMENTS

Condition of home
O Don't know
1 Good
2 Fair or average
3 Poor

Social adjustment of subject
O Don't know
1 Good
2 Fair or average
3 Poor

Cooperation of interviewee
O Don't know
1 Good
2 Fair or average
3 Poor

Reliability of answers
O Don't know
1 Good
2 Fair or average
3 Poor

*Other comments

How would you describe the discomfort or pain (worry for mental symptom) caused by this symptom?	How much inconvenience or disability does this symptom cause?	How serious do you think this symptom might be? A Not known B Not serious C Might be serious D Serious
Not known	Not known	A B C D
	None	A B C D
	Slight	A B C D
	Moderate	A B C D
	Severe	A B C D
None	Not known	A B C D
	None	A B C D
	Slight	A B C D
	Moderate	A B C D
	Severe	A B C D
Slight	Not known	A B C D
	None	A B C D
	Slight	A B C D
	Moderate	A B C D
	Severe	A B C D
Moderate	Not known	A B C D
	None	A B C D
	Slight	A B C D
	Moderate	A B C D
	Severe	A B C D
Severe	Not known	A B C D
	None	A B C D
	Slight	A B C D
	Moderate	A B C D
	Severe	A B C D

Did this symptom start during the past 2 weeks?	How long have you had this symptom? (or how frequently if episodic?)	Whom have you seen about this symptom? A Not known B Nobody C Family or relative D Friend or acquaintance E Nurse or health visitor F Dentist, chiropodist, optician (direct) G Own GP, partner or locum H Hospital doctor in casualty or out-patient (direct) I Other (code highest if more than one except other)
Not known	Not known	A B C D E F G H I
	2 days or less	A B C D E F G H I
Yes - and never had before	3 - 6 days	A B C D E F G H I
	7 - 14 days	A B C D E F G H I
	1 or 2 times	A B C D E F G H I
Yes - have had before, but new episode	3 - 6 times	A B C D E F G H I
	7 times or more	A B C D E F G H I
	2 - 12 weeks	A B C D E F G H I
No - started before this fortnight	3 - 12 months	A B C D E F G H I
	1 - 5 years	A B C D E F G H I
	More than 5 years	A B C D E F G H I

APPENDIX II

SYMPTOM PREVALENCE

PHYSICAL SYMPTOMS FOR ALL AGES (1,344 CASES)

Feeling more tired than usual or generally run-down		305 (22.7%)
(a) More tired than usual	216 (16.1%)	
(b) Generally run-down	22 (1.6%)	
(a) and (b)	67 (5.0%)	
A change in weight		117 (8.7%)
(a) Loss of weight (excluding deliberate dieting)	44 (3.3%)	
(b) Gain in weight (excluding pregnancy)	73 (5.4%)	
Fever, or unusual sweating or flushing		107 (8.0%)
(a) Fever	34 (2.5%)	
(b) Unusual sweating	30 (2.2%)	
(c) Unusual flushing	22 (1.6%)	
(a) and (b)	9 (0.7%)	
(b) and (c)	7 (0.5%)	
(a) and (c)	1 (0.1%)	
(a), (b) and (c)	4 (0.3%)	
Trouble with skin		204 (15.2%)
(a) Rash or irritation	167 (12.4%)	
(b) Sores or ulcers	11 (0.8%)	
(c) Boils or other skin trouble	23 (1.7%)	
(a) and (b)	1 (0.1%)	
(a) and (c)	2 (0.1%)	
Trouble with hair		68 (5.1%)
(a) Loss of hair	14 (1.0%)	
(b) Superfluous hair	O	
(c) Dandruff	54 (4.0%)	
Lumps under skin		65 (4.8%)
(a) Lumps or swollen glands (other than in breast)	57 (4.2%)	
(b) Swellings such as a rupture	6 (0.4%)	
(c) Lumps in breast	2 (0.1%)	
Change of colour in skin or in whites of eyes		22 (1.6%)
(a) Paler than usual	12 (0.9%)	
(b) Yellower than usual	3 (0.2%)	
(c) Other discolouration such as bruising	7 (0.5%)	

Feeling more thirsty than usual or cold apart from the
weather   76 (5.7%)
(a) More thirsty than usual   48 (3.6%)
(b) More cold apart from the weather   19 (1.4%)
(a) and (b)   9 (0.7%)
Change of appetite   106 (7.9%)
(a) Loss of appetite   70 (5.2%)
(b) Gain of appetite, or feeling hungry 36 (2.7%)
Trouble with teeth, or difficulty in eating or
swallowing   148 (11.0%)
(a) Trouble with teeth   105 (7.8%)
(b) Difficulty in eating because of mouth
    or gums   25 (1.9%)
(c) Difficulty in swallowing because of
    trouble in throat (or oesophagus)   12 (0.9%)
(a) and (b)   5 (0.4%)
(a) and (c)   1 (0.1%)
Nausea or vomiting   120 (8.9%)
(a) Nausea or feeling like vomiting   45 (3.3%)
(b) Retching without bringing up food   15 (1.1%)
(c) Vomiting up food or drink   59 (4.4%)
(d) Vomiting up blood which had not been
    swallowed   1 (0.1%)
Heartburn or indigestion   197 (14.7%)
(a) Heartburn   84 (6.3%)
(b) Indigestion   84 (6.3%)
(a) and (b)   29 (2.2%)
Other abdominal or tummy pain, or trouble with bowels   168 (12.5%)
(a) Pain in abdomen or tummy   69 (5.1%)
(b) Diarrhoea   23 (1.7%)
(c) Constipation   56 (4.2%)
(a) and (b)   10 (0.7%)
(a) and (c)   9 (0.7%)
(a), (b) and (c)   1 (0.1%)
Trouble with opening bowels   31 (2.3%)
(a) Pain on defaecation   15 (1.1%)
(b) Red blood on stool or paper   11 (0.8%)
(a) and (b)   5 (0.4%)
Difficulty or discomfort in passing water   29 (2.2%)
(a) More difficult than usual   10 (0.7%)
(b) Discomfort such as pain or burning   16 (1.2%)
(a) and (b)   3 (0.2%)
Passing water more often than usual   75 (5.6%)
(a) More frequently during the day   22 (1.6%)
(b) More frequently at night   24 (1.8%)
(a) and (b)   29 (2.2%)
Trouble with water coming away too quickly   32 (2.4%)
(a) Having to run to toilet   6 (0.4%)
(b) Leaks when straining, coughing or
    laughing   9 (0.7%)
(a) and (b)   17 (1.3%)
Unusual colour or smell about water   18 (1.3%)
(a) Strong smell   9 (0.7%)
(b) Reddish/brown discolouration   5 (0.4%)
(a) and (b)   4 (0.3%)

Pain or swelling in private parts or front passage   5 (0.4%)
(a) Pain   3 (0.2%)
(b) Swelling   2 (0.1%)
Discharge or irritation in private parts or front
passage   41 (3.1%)
(a) Discharge   21 (1.6%)
(b) Irritation   10 (0.7%)
(a) and (b)   10 (0.7%)
Trouble with periods   35 (2.6%)
(a) Pain with last period   20 (1.5%)
(b) Unusually heavy last period   10 (0.7%)
(c) Bleeding between periods, or post-
    menopausal   1 (0.1%)
(a) and (b)   4 (0.3%)
Irregularity or absence of period if pre-menopausal   41 (3.1%)
(a) Irregularity of periods   33 (2.5%)
(b) Absence of periods and probably not
    pregnant   2 (0.1%)
(c) Absence of periods and probably pregnant   6 (0.4%)
Trouble with pregnancy   10 (0.7%)
(a) Morning sickness   2 (0.1%)
(b) Pain or bleeding   1 (0.1%)
(c) Other   3 (0.2%)
(b) and (c)   1 (0.1%)
(a) and (c)   2 (0.1%)
(a), (b) and (c)   1 (0.1%)
Trouble with nose   365 (27.2%)
(a) Stuffy or runny nose, or catarrh at back
    of nose   355 (26.4%)
(b) Nose bleeds   8 (0.6%)
(a) and (b)   2 (0.1%)
Trouble with throat or voice   154 (11.5%)
(a) Sore throats   89 (6.6%)
(b) Hoarseness or loss of voice   49 (3.6%)
(c) Other   3 (0.2%)
(a) and (b)   12 (0.9%)
(b) and (c)   1 (0.1%)
Cough   376 (28.0%)
(a) Cough now, or during the past 2 weeks   214 (15.9%)
(b) Usually cough first on getting up   84 (6.3%)
(a) and (b)   78 (5.8%)
Phlegm   265 (19.7%)
(a) Phlegm now, or during the past 2 weeks   117 (8.7%)
(b) Usually phlegm first thing on getting
    up   87 (6.5%)
(a) and (b)   61 (4.5%)
Wheezing or coughing up blood   106 (7.9%)
(a) Chest sounding wheezy or whistling   53 (3.9%)
(b) Attacks of shortness of breath with
    wheezing   14 (1.0%)
(c) Coughing up blood which had not been
    swallowed   2 (0.1%)
(a) and (b)   34 (2.5%)
(a) and (c)   2 (0.1%)
(a), (b) and (c)   1 (0.1%)

Shortness of breath	260	(19.3%)
(a) When hurrying on level ground or walking up slight hill	166	(12.4%)
(b) When walking with people of own age on level ground	17	(1.3%)
(c) Having to stop for breath when walking at own pace on level ground	34	(2.5%)
(d) When washing or dressing	20	(1.5%)
(e) When sitting quietly	23	(1.7%)
Attacks of palpitations or breathlessness	101	(7.5%)
(a) Attacks of palpitations when heart beats fast for no apparent reason	61	(4.5%)
(b) Attacks of breathlessness when lying down	7	(0.5%)
(c) Sudden attacks of breathlessness when lying down at night	12	(0.9%)
(a) and (b)	3	(0.2%)
(b) and (c)	2	(0.1%)
(a) and (c)	5	(0.4%)
(a), (b) and (c)	11	(0.8%)
Ankle swelling or varicose veins	211	(15.7%)
(a) Ankle swelling in both ankles	62	(4.6%)
(b) Varicose veins	125	(9.3%)
(a) and (b)	24	(1.8%)
Pain or discomfort in chest which may go to arm	94	(7.0%)
(a) Comes on when walking and goes in 10 minutes or less if stop or slow down	25	(1.9%)
(b) Severe pain across front of chest which lasts for half an hour or more	17	(1.3%)
(a) and (b)	1	(0.1%)
(c) Other pain or discomfort in chest	51	(3.8%)
Pain in calf of either leg	114	(8.5%)
(a) Comes on when standing still or sitting	13	(1.0%)
(b) Comes on only when walking, and goes in 10 minutes or less if stand still	17	(1.3%)
(a) and (b)	3	(0.2%)
(c) Other pain in calf of either leg	81	(6.0%)
Any injuries during the past two weeks	124	(9.2%)
(a) Burn	15	(1.1%)
(b) Other minor injury or accident such as a fall with bruising	104	(7.7%)
(c) Other serious injury or accident such as fall with broken bone	5	(0.4%)
Trouble with joints	149	(11.1%)
(a) Pain, swelling, tenderness, or redness in small joints of hands or feet	48	(3.6%)
(b) Pain, swelling, tenderness or redness in large joints	63	(4.7%)
(c) Morning stiffness	9	(0.7%)
(a) and (b)	9	(0.7%)
(b) and (c)	4	(0.3%)
(a) and (c)	4	(0.3%)
(a), (b) and (c)	12	(0.9%)

Pain in spine or large bones		193 (14.4%)
(a) Low back pain	72 (5.4%)	
(b) Pain elsewhere in spine	33 (2.5%)	
(c) Pain in large bones	67 (5.0%)	
(a) and (b)	3 (0.2%)	
(b) and (c)	8 (0.6%)	
(a) and (c)	4 (0.3%)	
(a), (b) and (c)	6 (0.4%)	
Trouble with feet		283 (21.1%)
(a) Bunions, corns, or callosities	192 (14.3%)	
(b) Ingrowing toenails	19 (1.4%)	
(c) Flat feet or other	60 (4.5%)	
(a) and (b)	6 (0.4%)	
(b) and (c)	1 (0.1%)	
(a) and (c)	4 (0.3%)	
(a), (b) and (c)	1 (0.1%)	
Loss of consciousness or convulsions		21 (1.6%)
(a) Loss of consciousness or black-outs	16 (1.2%)	
(b) Convulsions or fits	5 (0.4%)	
Headaches or dizziness, or feeling more irritable and jumpy than usual		318 (23.7%)
(a) Headaches	174 (12.9%)	
(b) Spells of dizziness or vertigo	66 (4.9%)	
(c) Feeling more irritable and jumpy than usual	18 (1.3%)	
(a) and (b)	27 (2.0%)	
(b) and (c)	4 (0.3%)	
(a) and (c)	13 (1.0%)	
(a), (b) and (c)	16 (1.2%)	
Facial pain, loss of speech or balance		34 (2.6%)
(a) Pain in face for no apparent reason	9 (0.7%)	
(b) Loss of power of speech	6 (0.4%)	
(c) Loss of ability to balance on feet	16 (1.2%)	
(b) and (c)	2 (0.1%)	
(a), (b) and (c)	1 (0.1%)	
Trouble with ears		214 (15.9%)
(a) Pain, irritation or wax in ears	51 (3.8%)	
(b) Difficulty in hearing	110 (8.2%)	
(c) Ringing or buzzing in ears	18 (1.3%)	
(a) and (b)	14 (1.0%)	
(b) and (c)	8 (0.6%)	
(a) and (c)	6 (0.4%)	
(a), (b) and (c)	7 (0.5%)	
Trouble with eyes		205 (15.3%)
(a) Pain, irritation, or watering of eyes	85 (6.3%)	
(b) Difficulty in seeing	86 (6.4%)	
(c) Loss of sight in one or both eyes	16 (1.2%)	
(a) and (b)	14 (1.0%)	
(b) and (c)	1 (0.1%)	
(a) and (c)	3 (0.2%)	
Loss of power in limbs		27 (2.0%)
(a) Loss of power in upper limbs	11 (0.8%)	
(b) Loss of power in lower limbs	9 (0.7%)	
(a) and (b)	7 (0.5%)	

Loss of feeling or alteration of sensation in limbs   103 (7.7%)
(a) Loss of feeling, tingling or numbness
    in upper limbs   51 (3.8%)
(b) Loss of feeling, tingling or numbness
    in lower limbs   32 (2.4%)
(a) and (b)   20 (1.5%)

MENTAL SYMPTOMS FOR ADULTS (964 CASES)

Anxiety, fears, or loneliness   195 (20.2%)
(a) Feeling anxious at times without
    knowing the reason   120 (12.4%)
(b) Afraid of being in a wide open, or
    enclosed space   13 (1.3%)
(c) Feeling lonely   25 (2.6%)
(a) and (b)   8 (0.8%)
(b) and (c)   1 (0.1%)
(a) and (c)   24 (2.5%)
(a), (b) and (c)   4 (0.4%)
Sleeplessness   198 (20.5%)
(a) Difficulty in getting off to sleep
    without sleeping pills   113 (11.7%)
(b) Waking in the early hours and being
    unable to get off to sleep again
    without sleeping pills   38 (3.9%)
(a) and (b)   47 (4.9%)
Loss in interest in things   170 (17.6%)
(a) Losing interest in almost everything   35 (3.6%)
(b) Finding it difficult to concentrate   63 (6.5%)
(c) Being slower in everything you do   16 (1.7%)
(a) and (b)   15 (1.6%)
(b) and (c)   11 (1.1%)
(a) and (c)   1 (0.1%)
(a), (b) and (c)   29 (3.0%)
Worries about other people   83 (8.6%)
(a) People talking about you and criticizing
    you through no fault of your own   78 (8.1%)
(b) People trying to harm you through no
    fault of your own   1 (0.1%)
(a) and (b)   4 (0.4%)
Are you bothered about periods of excitability?   62 (6.4%)
(a) Times when exciting new ideas and
    schemes occur to you one after the
    other   42 (4.4%)
(b) Being so cheerful that you want to
    laugh and joke with everyone   10 (1.0%)
(a) and (b)   10 (1.0%)
Are you bothered by worries about doing things exactly
right?   124 (12.9%)
(a) Feeling you have to check things again
    and again, although you know there is
    really no need to   100 (10.4%)

(b) Having an uneasy feeling if you don't
do something in a certain order, or a
certain number of times   1 (0.1%)
(a) and (b)   23 (2.4%)
Feeling puzzled   46 (4.8%)
(a) Feeling puzzled, as if something had
gone wrong either with you or with the
world, without knowing just what it is 38 (3.9%)
(b) Hearing voices without knowing where
they come from   8 (0.8%)
Feeling low in spirits   196 (20.3%)
(a) Feeling so low in spirits that you just
sit for hours on end   161 (16.7%)
(b) Going to bed feeling you wouldn't care
if you never woke up   15 (1.6%)
(a) and (b)   20 (2.1%)

BEHAVIOURAL SYMPTOMS IN CHILDREN (380 CASES)

Do you think he or she is more difficult to manage than
others of the same age? (0-15 years)   33 (8.7%)
(a) Cries a lot or continually whining   5 (1.3%)
(b) Has real temper tantrums   4 (1.1%)
(c) Disobedient and/or sulky   7 (1.8%)
(a) and (b)   2 (0.5%)
(b) and (c)   8 (2.1%)
(a) and (c)   1 (0.3%)
(a), (b) and (c)   6 (1.6%)
Is there any other way in which he or she is more
difficult to manage than others of the same age?
(0-15 years)   27 (7.1%)
Not alert or not smiling (0-1 years)   0
Difficulty in sitting up on own or crawling (1-year-olds) 0
Difficulty in standing or walking on own (2-year-olds) 0
Difficulty in playing with other children (3-5 years) 3 (0.8%)
(a) Does not play well with other children
of the same age because always fighting
or quarrelling   1 (0.3%)
(b) Does not play well with other children
of the same age because shy and does not
have friends of the same age   2 (0.5%)
Difficulty with talking or sleeping (3-5 years)   14 (3.7%)
(a) Does not talk as well as he or she
should for age   3 (0.8%)
(b) Restless in sleep - tosses and turns -
wakes in the night - has frightening
dreams   7 (1.8%)
(c) Other   2 (0.5%)
(b) and (c)   2 (0.5%)
Difficulty with friends or at school (6-10 years) 17 (4.5%)
(a) Difficulty in making and keeping
friends   5 (1.3%)

(b) Difficulty in school work or learning
    to read compared with other children
    of same age   9 (2.4%)
(c) Other   0
(a) and (b)   2 (0.5%)
(a) and (c)   1 (0.3%)
Bed-wetting (6-10 years)   17 (4.5%)
(a) Occasionally   8 (2.1%)
(b) Sometimes   4 (1.1%)
(c) Frequently, or most nights   5 (1.3%)
Difficulty with friends or at school (11-15 years)   13 (3.4%)
(a) Difficulty in making and keeping
    friends   5 (1.3%)
(b) Difficulty with school work compared
    with children of same age   6 (1.6%)
(c) Other   0
(a) and (b)   1 (0.3%)
(a), (b) and (c)   1 (0.3%)
Getting into trouble (11-15 years)   6 (1.6%)
(a) Gets into trouble a lot at school
    (include truancy)   0
(b) Gets into trouble a lot outside school   5 (1.3%)
(c) Other   0
(a) and (c)   1 (0.3%)

SOCIAL SYMPTOMS FOR ADULTS (964 CASES)

Are there any difficulties with children or teenagers
which have been troubling you during the past two weeks? 49 (5.1%)
(a) Worry and/or inconvenience caused:
    None or not known   5 (0.5%)
    Slight   19 (2.0%)
    Moderate   7 (0.7%)
    A lot   18 (1.9%)
(b) Who was involved?
    Not known   1 (0.1%)
    Son(s)   26 (2.7%)
    Daughter(s)   17 (1.8%)
    Son(s) and daughter(s)   4 (0.4%)
    Granddaughter(s)   1 (0.1%)
(c) What age?
    Not known   6 (0.6%)
    0-1 years   0
    1-2 years   4 (0.4%)
    3-5 years   4 (0.4%)
    6-10 years   11 (1.1%)
    11-15 years   3 (0.3%)
    16 to <20 years   10 (1.0%)
    Combination   11 (1.1%)
(d) Nature of difficulty
    Not known   1 (0.1%)
    Not getting on with parents   5 (0.5%)
    Behavioural disorder   17 (1.8%)

Truancy   1 (0.1%)
Trouble with authorities (other than
truancy)   4 (0.4%)
Mental handicap   2 (0.2%)
Illness   8 (0.8%)
Other   3 (0.3%)
Combination   8 (0.8%)
Are there any difficulties with other members of the
family or relatives (other than children and teenagers)
which have been troubling you during the past two weeks? 68 (7.1%)
(a) Worry and/or inconvenience caused:
    None or not known   4 (0.4%)
    Slight   21 (2.2%)
    Moderate   14 (1.5%)
    A lot   29 (3.0%)
(b) Who was involved?
    Not known   2 (0.2%)
    Spouse   16 (1.7%)
    Sib(s) (and in-law)   11 (1.1%)
    Parent(s)   13 (1.3%)
    Parent(s)-in-law   3 (0.3%)
    Grandparent(s) (and in-law)   1 (0.1%)
    Children   16 (1.7%)
    Aunt(s) and uncle(s)   1 (0.1%)
    Other   2 (0.2%)
    Combination   3 (0.3%)
(c) What age and sex?
    Not known   4 (0.4%)
    Male - 0-15 years   1 (0.1%)
           16-44 years   18 (1.9%)
           45-64 years   7 (0.7%)
           65+   0
    Female - 0-15 years   0
             16-44 years   8 (0.8%)
             45-64 years   9 (0.9%)
             65+   11 (1.1%)
    Combination   10 (1.0%)
(d) Nature of difficulty
    Not known   2 (0.2%)
    Illness (other than alcohol)   13 (1.3%)
    Personal relationships   24 (2.5%)
    Dependent relative(s)   6 (0.6%)
    Alcohol   7 (0.6%)
    Other   10 (1.0%)
    Combination   6 (0.6%)
Are there any financial difficulties which have been
troubling you during the past two weeks?   93 (9.6%)
(a) Worry and/or inconvenience caused
    None or not known   8 (0.8%)
    Slight   35 (3.6%)
    Moderate   19 (2.0%)
    A lot   31 (3.2%)

(b) Income difficulties

None or not known	40	(4.1%)
Not enough income (no specific reason)	5	(0.5%)
On strike ≤2 weeks or unknown	3	(0.3%)
On strike known to be >2 weeks	4	(0.4%)
Unemployed ≤1 year or unknown	16	(1.7%)
Unemployed >1 year	6	(0.6%)
Pension	3	(0.3%)
Ill health	7	(0.7%)
Other (e.g. on short time)	5	(0.5%)
Combination	4	(0.4%)

(c) Expenditure difficulties

None or not known	33	(3.4%)
Not enough to spend (no specific reason)	15	(1.6%)
Difficulty in handling money	1	(0.1%)
Rent and rates	14	(1.5%)
Power bills	3	(0.3%)
Hire purchase	1	(0.1%)
Other specific bills	13	(1.3%)
Other	2	(0.2%)
Combination	11	(1.1%)

Are there any other difficulties or problems with day-to-
day life which have been troubling you during the past
two weeks?   103 (10.7%)

(a) Worry or inconvenience caused

None or not known	13	(1.3%)
Slight	35	(3.6%)
Moderate	27	(2.8%)
A lot	28	(2.9%)

(b) Nature of difficulty

Not known	0	
Disability or illness	14	(1.5%)
Bereavement	3	(0.3%)
Children	5	(0.5%)
Work	9	(0.9%)
Unemployment	9	(0.9%)
Housing	33	(3.4%)
Legal or crime	8	(0.8%)
Other	12	(1.2%)
Combination	10	(1.0%)

(c) Duration of difficulty

Not known	64	(6.6%)
<2 weeks	4	(0.4%)
2 to <4 weeks	2	(0.2%)
1 to <3 months	7	(0.7%)
3 to <12 months	12	(1.2%)
1 to <5 years	13	(1.3%)
5 to <10 years	1	(0.1%)

APPENDIX III
REFERRAL BEHAVIOUR

TABLE III.1   Referral of physical symptoms by number of subjects

Number of physical symptoms referred by each subject	Not known	Nobody	Family or relative	Friend or acquaintance	Nurse or health visitor	Dentist, chiropodist, optician (direct)	Own GP, partner or locum	Hospital doctor in Casualty or Outpatients (direct)	Other
1	9	271	100	8	9	129	225	55	59
2		217	38	3		3	117	6	6
3		154	16	1			85	1	1
4		98	14	1	1		45		
5		66	7				33		
6		58	8				25		
7		38	5				20		
8		24	2				12		
9		14	5				10		
10		8	1				3		
11		8	2				7		
12		6					1		
13+		5	4				3		
Total number of subjects	9	967	202	13	10	132	586	62	66
% of all subjects	1%	72%	15%	1%	1%	10%	44%	5%	5%

(Percentages out of 1,344 subjects)

TABLE III.2 Referral of mental symptoms by number of adults

Number of mental symptoms referred by each adult	Not known	Nobody	Family or relative	Friend or acquaintance	Nurse or health visitor	Dentist, chiropodist, optician (direct)	Own GP, partner or locum	Hospital doctor in Casualty or Outpatients (direct)	Other
1	3	221	41	8			83	2	1
2		107	14				26		
3		61	6				13		
4		20	5				1		
5		6							
6		5							
7			1						
Total number of subjects	3	420	67	8	0	0	123	2	1
% of all adults	–	44%	7%	1%	–	–	13%	–	–

(Percentages out of 964 adults)

TABLE III.3 Referral of behavioural symptoms by number of children

Number of behavioural symptoms referred for each child	Not known	Nobody	Family or relative	Friend or acquaintance	Nurse or health visitor	Dentist, chiropodist, optician (direct)	Own GP, partner or locum	Hospital doctor in Casualty or Outpatients (direct)	other
1	1	44	7				18		11
2		6	4				1		5
3		2	2						1
Total number of children	1	52	13	0	0	0	19	0	17
% of all children	–	14%	3%	–	–	–	5%	–	4%

(Percentages out of 380 children)

TABLE III.4   Informal referral of social symptoms by number of adults

Number of social symptoms referred by each adult	Not known or none*	Nothing because felt powerless or helpless	Nothing because of other specific reason	Avoidance	Self	Informal through relative	Informal through friend	Informal through other or combination of informal
1	1	11	15	3	68	16	5	2
2	12	2						
3	97							
Total number of adults	110	13	15	3	68	16	5	2
% of all adults	11%	1%	2%	–	7%	2%	1%	–

(Percentages out of 964 adults)

*[Most of those coded as 'not known or none' for informal referrals, had made a formal referral instead]

TABLE III.5 Formal referral of social symptoms by number of adults

Number of social symptoms referred by each adult	Not known or none*	Doctor/hospital	Nurse or health visitor	Social Worker/social work dept/ medical social worker	Teacher	Minister	Factor/housing dept	Social security/employment exchange	Other formal	Combination
1	3	27	1	8	2	1	15	32	16	14
2	11							2	1	1
3	93									
Total number of adults	107	27	1	8	2	1	15	34	17	15
% of all adults	11%	3%	–	1%	–	–	2%	4%	2%	2%

(Percentages out of 964 adults)

*[Most of those coded 'not known or none' for formal referrals, had made an informal referral instead]

APPENDIX IV CORRELATIONS

Dependent

Independent variable	Symptom frequencies			
	Physical	Mental	Behavioural	Social
Practice				
Month				
Age				
Sex				
Age-sex groups				
Marital status				
Employment status				
Social class				
Education				
Religion				
Housing tenure				
Period when house built				
Type of house				
Number of rooms				
Number of occupants				
Density				
Toilet facilities				
Hot water and bath/shower				
Amenities				
Years in present residence				
Years with present GP				
Previous residence				
Mother's residence at birth				
Main place of upbringing				
Birth and upbringing				
Number of moves				
Relatives seen in past week				

variables						Number of
Tendency to refer		'Iceberg'		'Trivia'		significant
Medical	Social	Medical	Social	Medical	Social	correlations
						-
						-
						10
						2
						11
						7
						15
						1
						5
						5
						4
						1
						3
						5
						5
						3
						1
						1
						-
						2
						7
						6
						2
						3
						3
						8
						1

	Dependent			
	Symptom frequencies			
Independent variable	Physical	Mental	Behavioural	Social
Number of previous illnesses	▨	▨		
Number of short hospital stays	▨	▨		▨
Number of long hospital stays	▨			
Experience of doctors and hospitals		▨		▨
Self-estimate of present health	▨	▨		▨
Present illnesses or disabilities	▨	▨	▨	▨
Smoking habits	▨	▨	✕	
Smoking history	▨		✕	
Number of cigarettes per day	▨		✕	
Smoking score	▨			
Interviewee relationship			▨	✕
Age of interviewee		✕	✕	✕
Sex of interviewee		✕	✕	✕
Personality-extroversion			▨	✕
Personality-neuroticism	▨			▨
Intelligence				
Surgery visits in past year	▨	▨		
Home visits by GP in past year	▨	▨		
Preference for health centre				
Suggested improvements		▨		▨
Social worker seen in past year	▨	▨		▨
Why social worker seen	▨			
Problems social worker deals with				
Anyone else to social worker - who?		▨		▨
Anyone else to social worker - why?				
Other helping agencies - which?	▨			▨
Other helping agencies - why?	▨			▨

variables						Number of
Tendency to refer		'Iceberg'		'Trivia'		significant
Medical	Social	Medical	Social	Medical	Social	correlations
▨		▨				7
▨		▨		▨		10
			▨			2
				▨	▨	6
▨		▨		▨		12
▨			▨	▨		13
▨						3
▨						2
▨		▨	▨	▨		8
▨						2
	✕		✕		✕	1
	✕		✕		✕	–
	✕		✕		✕	–
					▨	3
		▨	▨	▨		10
			▨			1
▨		▨		▨		9
▨	▨		▨			6
			▨			1
					▨	3
▨			▨	▨		9
						1
▨					▨	2
			▨			3
						–
	▨	▨			▨	7
		▨				6

Independent variable	Dependent			
	Symptom frequencies			
	Physical	Mental	Behavioural	Social
How doctor contacted	▨			
Difficulty in contacting doctor	▨	▨		▨
Travel to health centre	▨	▨		▨
Minutes to health centre	▨			
Travel/time to health centre		▨		▨
How to contact social worker	▨		▨	▨
Nearest social work dept		▨		▨
Medical knowledge score				
Neighbourhood advice			▨	▨
Action if in doubt				▨
Home remedies				
Which doctor preferred to see first			▨	
Prescribed medicine taking	▨	▨		▨
Number of prescribed medicines	▨	▨		▨
Unprescribed medicine taking	▨	▨	▨	▨
Number of unprescribed medicines	▨	▨	▨	▨
Method of contraception			▨	▨
Contraceptive advice				▨
Contraceptive supplies				
Contraceptive facilities				
Other personal matters	▨	▨	▨	
Comments on interview	▨	▨	▨	
Length of interview	▨	▨	▨	▨
Others present at interview	▨			
Condition of home		▨		▨
Social adjustment	▨	▨	▨	▨
Cooperation				

variables						Number of
Tendency to refer		'Iceberg'		'Trivia'		significant
Medical	Social	Medical	Social	Medical	Social	correlations
						3
						5
						5
						1
						3
						6
						4
						-
						2
						1
						-
						3
						11
						14
						9
						9
						3
						1
						-
						-
						5
						11
						13
						7
						6
						10
						1

	Dependent			
Independent variable	Symptom frequencies			
	Physical	Mental	Behavioural	Social
Reliability	▨	▨		▨
Mean pain score		◺	◺	
Mean disability score				
Mean seriousness score				
Mean duration score	▨	▨	▨	▨
Mean worry score		◺	◺	
Physical symptom frequency	⊠	▨	▨	▨
Mental symptom frequency	▨	⊠	⊠	▨
Behavioural symptom frequency	▨	⊠	⊠	⊠
Social symptom frequency	▨	▨	⊠	⊠
Mean medical referral	▨	▨	⊠	⊠
Mean social referral	▨	⊠	⊠	▨
Medical symptom 'Iceberg'	▨	▨	⊠	⊠
Social symptom 'Iceberg'	▨	◺	⊠	▨
Medical symptom 'Trivia'	▨	◺	⊠	▨
Social symptom 'Trivia'	◺		⊠	▨
Number of significant correlations	95	72	19	65

☐   No significant correlations

▨   Difference between means significant at 0.05 level on breakdown

◺   Chi-squared test significant at 0.05 level on cross-tabulation

▨   Both difference between means and chi-squared test significant at 0.05 level

⊠   Correlations not done as inappropriate

The independent variables are given in the order in which they appear in the questionnaire (Appendix I), with computed variables either next to the variables from which they were derived, or at the end in the case of the grading scales, symptom frequencies and referral scores.

variables						Number of
Tendency to refer		'Iceberg'		'Trivia'		significant
Medical	Social	Medical	Social	Medical	Social	correlations
						5
						8
						7
						4
						13
						7
						13
						12
						1
						13
						10
						7
						11
						8
						6
						4
55	10	77	26	62	19	500

APPENDIX V

MULTIPLE REGRESSION

The following tables show the results of the multiple regression analysis for each dependent variable in turn. The results are tabulated by listing the independent variables in order of the values of the standardized regression coefficients. This order is not necessarily the same as the order in which the variables were entered into the regression equation, for two reasons. First, because the predictive value of the next independent variable to be entered depended on its unstandardized regression coefficient; this differed from the standardized regression coefficient because the latter takes into account differences in the scales used, so that the values for each independent variable can be compared. The second reason why the rank order of the standardized regression coefficient did not necessarily reflect the sequence of steps in the equation was that the interaction effects of subsequent variables might alter the regression coefficients of those variables already entered. The values of the regression coefficients given therefore only relate to the final step of the equation and reflect the inter-action of all the variables added.

Those independent variables for which the unstandardized regres-sion coefficients were significant at the 0.05 level in the final step of the equation, are underlined in the tables. Because of the effect of standardizing the regression coefficients a variable which was not significant in this way was occasionally ranked above a variable for which the unstandardized regression coefficient was significant. In addition to the standardized regression coefficients, the change in variance produced by each independent variable as it was entered into the regression equation is also tabulated. The regression coefficients and changes in variance are given corrected to three places of decimals, so that very small changes in variance appear as zero. Although such variables had negligible effect upon the overall linear regression for the dependent variable, the amount of change produced satisfied the minimal default values for inclu-sion in the regression equation. Variables which did not have significant correlation coefficients are shown in the tables in order to indicate those factors for which the interaction effects had been taken into account. The direction in which the independent variables affected the linear regression is indicated in brackets after each variable, except where it is implicit for positive correlations that the dependent variable increased directly with the independent variable.

TABLE V.1   Multiple regression for frequency of physical symptoms

Independent variable	Standardized regression coefficient	Change in variance
Neuroticism score	0.223	0.061
Number of short hospital stays	0.218	0.178
Age	0.191	0.041
Number of moves	0.107	0.011
Number of cigarettes smoked	0.091	0.004
Religion (passive allegiance)	0.077	0.009
Sex (female)	0.067	0.004
Birth and upbringing (away from Glasgow)	0.056	0.002
Intelligence score (low)	-0.005	0.004
Number of previous illnesses	0.055	0.002
House ownership (tenant)	-0.050	0.002
Previous residence (in Glasgow)	-0.045	0.002
Basic amenities (lack of)	0.039	0.001
Number of long hospital stays	0.033	0.001
High rise flats (living in)	0.032	0.001
Separation or divorce	0.029	0.001
Years in present residence (few)	-0.025	0.000
Unemployment - not due to illness	0.025	0.000
Density (low)	-0.019	0.000
Contacts with relatives (few)	-0.014	0.000
Age of housing (recent)	0.012	0.000

TABLE V.2 Multiple regression for frequency of mental symptoms

Independent variable	Standardized regression coefficient	Change in variance
Neuroticism score	0.348	0.157
Number of short hospital stays	0.119	0.031
Sex (female)	0.106	0.006
Age of housing (older)	-0.096	0.003
Unemployment - not due to illness	0.091	0.006
Age	0.085	0.006
Intelligence score (low)	-0.082	0.014
Religion (passive allegiance)	0.075	0.005
Social class (lower)	0.074	0.002
High rise flats (living in)	0.069	0.004
Number of previous illnesses	0.066	0.002
Birth and upbringing (in Glasgow)	-0.058	0.002
Contacts with relatives (few)	-0.054	0.003
Years in present residence (few)	-0.053	0.002
Basic amenities (present)	-0.051	0.002
Previous residence (away from Glasgow)	0.049	0.002
Density (low)	-0.049	0.003
Separation or divorce	0.027	0.001
House ownership (tenant)	-0.024	0.000
Number of long hospital stays (few)	-0.019	0.000

TABLE V.3   Multiple regression for frequency of behavioural
            symptoms

Independent variable	Standardized regression coefficient	Change in variance
Number of long hospital stays	0.300	0.090
Relationship of respondent (not a parent)	0.125	0.016
Neuroticism score of respondent	0.109	0.014
Religion (passive allegiance)	0.067	0.004
Sex (male)	-0.061	0.006
Number of short hospital stays	0.061	0.003
Sex of respondent (female)	0.041	0.001
High rise flats (living in)	0.038	0.001
Intelligence score of respondent	0.029	0.001
Birth and upbringing (away from Glasgow)	0.027	0.001
Density	0.023	0.000
House ownership (owner occupier)	0.020	0.001
Social class (higher)	-0.018	0.000

TABLE V.4 Multiple regression for frequency of social symptoms

Independent variable	Standardized regression coefficient	Change in variance
Neuroticism score	0.191	0.051
Unemployment - not due to illness	0.174	0.028
Age	0.135	0.005
Separation or divorce	0.114	0.015
Number of short hospital stays	0.113	0.011
High rise flats (not living in)	-0.079	0.005
Religion (passive allegiance)	0.072	0.006
Years in present residence (few)	-0.070	0.004
Density	0.062	0.001
Contacts with relatives (few)	-0.052	0.002
Birth and upbringing (in Glasgow)	-0.052	0.002
Number of previous illnesses (few)	-0.046	0.002
Basic amenities (present)	-0.042	0.001
Age of housing (older)	-0.039	0.001
Intelligence score	0.034	0.001
Sex (female)	0.033	0.001
Number of cigarettes smoked	0.033	0.001
Number of moves	0.020	0.000
Social class (higher)	-0.018	0.001

TABLE V.5   Multiple regression for tendency to refer medical
            symptoms formally

Independent variable	Standardized regression coefficient	Change in variance
Number of present illnesses	0.207	0.056
Mean seriousness score	0.154	0.021
Age (younger)	-0.132	0.006
Mean pain score	0.116	0.045
Self-estimate of present health (poor)	0.095	0.005
Mean disability score	0.084	0.004
Birth and upbringing (away from Glasgow)	0.081	0.004
Difficulty in contacting doctor	0.080	0.005
Neuroticism score (low)	-0.068	0.003
High rise flats (living in)	0.063	0.004
Unemployment - not due to illness (absence of)	-0.061	0.005
Previous residence (in Glasgow)	-0.058	0.002
Doctor preference (own doctor or partner)	-0.055	0.004
Sex (female)	0.052	0.003
Preference for health centre	0.051	0.003
Number of previous illnesses (few)	-0.030	0.001
Experience of doctors and hospitals (poor)	-0.024	0.000
Mean duration score	0.022	0.000
Intelligence score (low)	-0.022	0.000
Number of moves	0.022	0.000
Religion (active allegiance)	-0.021	0.000
Contacting doctor by telephone	0.020	0.000
Years in present residence (few)	-0.018	0.000
Separation or divorce	0.016	0.000
Basic amenities (lack of)	0.014	0.000
Walking to health centre (absence of)	-0.014	0.000
Social class (lower)	0.013	0.000
Number of long hospital stays (few)	-0.011	0.000
Density (low)	-0.009	0.000
Contacts with relatives	0.007	0.000

TABLE V.6   Multiple regression for tendency to refer social
            symptoms formally

Independent variable	Standardized regression coefficient	Change in variance
Neuroticism score (low)	−0.275	0.037
Number of previous illnesses	0.269	0.041
Basic amenities (lack of)	0.203	0.035
Self-estimate of present health (poor)	0.130	0.008
Number of long hospital stays (few)	−0.118	0.012
Number of moves (few)	−0.103	0.011
Sex (female)	0.092	0.006
Years in present residence (few)	−0.086	0.007
Knowledge about contacting social worker (correct)	0.085	0.005
Previous residence (away from Glasgow)	0.080	0.004
High rise flats (living in)	0.064	0.003
Social class (lower)	0.060	0.003
Number of present illnesses (few)	−0.058	0.003
Knowledge about others contacting social worker (none)	−0.054	0.002
Density (low)	−0.046	0.001
Age (younger)	−0.040	0.001
Unemployment − not due to illness	0.035	0.001
Number of short hospital stays (few)	−0.034	0.001
Mean worry score	0.028	0.001
Religion (passive allegiance)	0.026	0.001

TABLE V.7   Multiple regression for medical symptom 'iceberg'

Independent variable	Standardized regression coefficient	Change in variance
Neuroticism score	0.189	0.030
Number of previous illnesses	0.169	0.054
Self-estimate of present health (poor)	0.125	0.013
Age	0.107	0.027
Number of moves	0.066	0.003
Sex (female)	0.058	0.002
Intelligence score (low)	-0.052	0.003
Walking to health centre (absence of)	-0.050	0.002
Time to health centre	0.040	0.001
Unemployment - not due to illness	0.034	0.002
Number of short hospital stays (few)	-0.032	0.001
Contact with relatives	0.032	0.001
Religion (passive allegiance)	0.031	0.001
Separation or divorce (absence of)	-0.029	0.001
Difficulty in contacting doctor (absence of)	-0.029	0.001
Density	0.028	0.001
Contacting doctor by telephone (absence of)	-0.021	0.000
Experience of doctors and hospitals (good)	0.018	0.000
Birth and upbringing (away from Glasgow)	0.016	0.000
Preference for health centre (absence of)	-0.016	0.000
Doctor preference (any doctor)	0.015	0.000
Number of long hospital stays	0.013	0.000
High rise flats (not living in)	-0.013	0.000
Previous residence (in Glasgow)	-0.011	0.000
Social class (lower)	0.009	0.000

TABLE V.8 Multiple regression for social symptom 'iceberg'

Independent variable	Standardized regression coefficient	Change in variance
Number of previous illnesses (few)	-0.118	0.005
Neuroticism score	0.107	0.013
Unemployment - not due to illness	0.075	0.005
Age	0.075	0.001
Knowledge about others contacting social worker	0.072	0.004
Number of short hospital stays	0.059	0.002
Number of present illnesses	0.056	0.003
High rise flats (not living in)	-0.055	0.002
Separation or divorce (absence of)	-0.049	0.002
Knowledge about nearest social work department (correct)	0.047	0.001
Knowledge about contacting social worker (wrong)	-0.044	0.001
Intelligence score	0.044	0.002
Density	0.041	0.001
Birth and upbringing (in Glasgow)	-0.037	0.001
Contacts with relatives (few)	-0.037	0.001
Basic amenities (present)	-0.037	0.001
Number of long hospital stays	0.030	0.001
Social class (higher)	-0.029	0.001
Years in present residence (few)	-0.028	0.000
Self-estimate of present health (poor)	0.019	0.000
Previous residence (in Glasgow)	-0.019	0.000

TABLE V.9   Multiple regression for medical symptom 'trivia'

Independent variable	Standardized regression coefficient	Change in variance
Number of present illnesses	0.169	0.038
Separation or divorce	0.115	0.015
Age	0.107	0.002
Experience of doctors and hospitals (poor)	-0.100	0.008
Years in present residence (few)	-0.086	0.006
Difficulty in contacting doctor	0.077	0.006
Number of short hospital stays	0.077	0.002
Sex (female)	0.070	0.006
Number of long hospital stays (few)	-0.058	0.003
Birth and upbringing (away from Glasgow)	0.052	0.001
Self-estimate of present health (good)	-0.049	0.001
Contacting doctor by telephone	0.047	0.002
Number of previous illnesses (few)	-0.044	0.001
Number of moves	0.042	0.008
Time to health centre	0.035	0.001
High rise flats (living in)	0.033	0.003
Religion (passive allegiance)	0.029	0.001
Social class (lower)	0.027	0.001
Previous residence (in Glasgow)	-0.027	0.001
Unemployment - not due to illness	0.027	0.001
Intelligence score	0.025	0.000
Density (low)	-0.016	0.000
Basic amenities (lack of)	0.013	0.000
Neuroticism score (low)	-0.010	0.000

TABLE V.10   Multiple regression for social symptom 'trivia'

Independent variable	Standardized regression coefficient	Change in variance
High rise flats (living in)	0.088	0.007
Number of present illnesses	0.088	0.009
Birth and upbringing (in Glasgow)	-0.071	0.002
Unemployment - not due to illness	0.062	0.003
Number of short hospital stays	0.061	0.001
Density	0.043	0.001
Intelligence score	0.041	0.001
Religion (active allegiance)	-0.040	0.002
Age	0.039	0.001
Number of previous illnesses (few)	-0.037	0.001
Number of long hospital stays	0.037	0.001
Previous residence (away from Glasgow)	0.030	0.001
Neuroticism score (low)	-0.029	0.001
Sex (female)	0.023	0.000
Social class (higher)	-0.023	0.000
Knowledge about others contacting social worker (none)	-0.022	0.000
Basic amenities (lack of)	0.020	0.000
Knowledge about contacting social worker (correct)	0.019	0.000
Years in present residence (few)	-0.017	0.000
Contacts with relatives (few)	-0.015	0.000
Separation or divorce (absence of)	-0.014	0.000

BIBLIOGRAPHY

Berger, P.L. (1967), 'Invitation to Sociology', Penguin, Harmonds-worth.

Bevan, J.M. and Draper, G.J. (1967), 'Appointment Systems in General Practice', Oxford University Press, London.

Blalock, M.M. (1972), 'Social Statistics', McGraw-Hill, Kogakusha Ltd, Tokyo.

Bloom, S. (1963), 'The Doctor and His Patient', Russel Sage Foundation, New York.

Bodenham, K.E. and Wellman, F. (1972), 'Foundation for Health Service Management', Scientific Control Systems, London.

Bowlby, J. (1965), 'Child Care and the Growth of Love', Penguin, Harmondsworth.

British Sociological Association and Social Science Research Council (1969), 'Comparability in Social Science', Heinemann, London.

Butterfield, W.J.H. (1968), 'Priorities in Medical Care', Nuffield Provincial Hospitals Trust, London.

Cartwright, A. (1967), 'Patients and Their Doctors - A Study of General Practice', Routledge & Kegan Paul, London.

Cartwright, A. (1970), 'Parents and Family Planning Services', Routledge & Kegan Paul, London.

Central Statistical Office (1973), 'Social Trends No.4', HMSO, London.

Corporation of the City of Glasgow (1972), Report of the Medical Officer of Health, Glasgow.

Department of Social Administration Edinburgh (1968), 'Social Work in Scotland', University of Edinburgh.

Documenta Geigy (1970), 'Scientific Tables', J.R. Geigy, Switzerland.

Dubos, R. (1959), 'The Mirage of Health', Allen & Unwin, London.

Dubos, R. (1965), 'Man Adapting', Yale University Press, New Haven and London.

Dunnell, K. and Cartwright, A. (1972), 'Medicine Takers, Prescribers and Hoarders', Routledge & Kegan Paul, London.

Durkheim, E. (1951), 'Suicide - A Study in Sociology', Glencoe Press, Riverside, N.J.

English, J. and Norman, P. (1974), 'One Hundred Years of Slum Clearance in England and Wales Policies and Programmes, 1868-1970', Discussion Papers in Social Research No.1, University of Glasgow.

English, J. and Norman, P. (1974), 'An Appraisal of Slum Clearance Procedures in England and Wales', Discussion Papers in Social Research No.4, University of Glasgow.

Forbes, J. (1974), 'Studies in Social Science and Planning', Scottish Academic Press, Edinburgh.

Gordon, G. (1966), 'Role, Theory and Illness', College and University Press, New Haven, Connecticut.

Hicks, D. (1977), 'Primary Health Care - A Review', Department of Health and Social Security, HMSO, London.

Hollingsworth, T.H. (1970), 'Migration: A Study Based on Scottish Experience', Oliver & Boyd, Edinburgh.

Holtermann, S. (1975), 'Census Indicators of Urban Deprivation', Working Note No.6, Department of the Environment, London.

Jefferys, M. (1965), 'An Anatomy of Social Welfare Services', Michael Joseph, London.

Jephcott, P. (1971), 'Homes in High Flats', Oliver & Boyd, Edinburgh.

Jones, F.A. (1972), 'Richard Asher Talking Sense', Pitman Medical, London.

Klein, D.C. (1968), 'Community Dynamics and Mental Health', John Wiley, New York.

Koos, E.L. (1954), 'The Health of Regionville', Columbia University Press, New York.

Martin, J.P. (1957), 'Social Aspects of Prescribing', Heinemann, London.

Mayer, J.E. and Timms, N. (1970), 'The Client Speaks', Routledge & Kegan Paul, London.

Merton, R.K. (1975), 'Social Theory and Social Structure', Glencoe Press, Riverside, N.J.

Moser, C.A. and Kalton, G. (1971), 'Survey Methods in Social Investigation', Heinemann Educational, London.

Nie, N.H., Bent, D.H. and Hull, C.H. (1970), 'Statistical Package for the Social Sciences', McGraw-Hill, New York.

Office of Health Economics (1968), 'General Practice Today', OHE, London.

Office of Health Economics (1972), 'Medicine and Society', OHE, London.

Office of Health Economics (1964), 'New Frontiers in Health', OHE, London.

Office of Health Economics (1973), 'Rheumatism and Arthritis in Britain', OHE, London.

Office of Health Economics (1973), 'Skin Disorders', OHE, London.

Office of Health Economics (1974), 'The Work of Primary Medical Care', OHE, London.

Office of Health Economics (1968), 'Without Prescription', OHE, London.

Office of Population Censuses and Surveys (1973), 'The General Household Survey', HMSO, London.

Parsons, T. (1951), 'The Social System', Routledge & Kegan Paul, London.

Pearse, I.H. and Crocker, L.H. (1943), 'The Peckham Experiment', Allen & Unwin, London.

Robinson, D. (1971), 'The Process of Becoming Ill', Routledge & Kegan Paul, London.

Royal College of Physicians (1971), 'Smoking and Health Now', Pitman Medical Scientific, London.

Royal College of General Practitioners (1972), 'The Future General
Practitioner: Learning and Teaching', British Medical Journal,
London.
Scottish Housing Advisory Committee (1967), 'Scotland's Older
Housing', Scottish Development Department, Edinburgh.
Scottish Housing Advisory Committee (1970), 'Council House Commun-
ities', Scottish Development Department, Edinburgh.
Silver, G.A. (1963), 'Family Medical Care', Harvard University Press,
Massachusetts.
Statistical Package for Social Sciences (1973), 'Update Manual',
Edinburgh University Press.
Susser, M. (1973), 'Causal Thinking in the Health Services', Oxford
University Press.
Timms, N. (1967), 'A Sociological Approach to Social Problems',
Routledge & Kegan Paul, London.
Timms, N. (1970), 'Social Work', Routledge & Kegan Paul, London.
Wadsworth, M.E.J., Butterfield, W.J.H. and Blaney, R. (1971),
'Health and Sickness: The Choice of Treatment', Tavistock, London.
Wootton, B. (1959), 'Social Science and Social Pathology', Allen &
Unwin, London.

INDEX

211